Concise Medical Textbooks

Pathology

Concise Medical Textbooks

Pathology

J. R. Tighe

BSc, MD, FRCP, FRCPE, FRCPath
Professor of Histopathology,
United Medical and Dental Schools of
Guy's and St Thomas' Hospitals
and Honorary Consultant Pathologist,
St Thomas' Hospital, London

D. R. Davies

AKC, MB, BS, MRCS, LRCP, FRCPath
Senior Lecturer in Histopathology,
United Medical and Dental Schools of
Guy's and St Thomas' Hospitals
and Honorary Consultant Pathologist,
St Thomas' Hospital, London

Fourth Edition

Baillière Tindall
London Philadelphia Toronto
Sydney Tokyo

Baillière Tindall   24–28 Oval Road
W.B. Saunders   London NW1 7DX

The Curtis Center, Independence Square West,
Philadelphia, PA 19106–3399, USA

55 Horner Avenue,
Toronto, Ontario M8Z 4X6, Canada

Harcourt Brace Jovanovich (Australia) Pty Ltd,
32-52 Smidmore Street, Marrickville, NSW 2204, Australia

Harcourt Brace Jovanovich Japan Inc.
Ichibancho Central Building, 22-1 Ichibancho
Chiyoda-ku, Tokyo 102, Japan

First edition 1964
Second edition 1967
Third edition 1972
Fourth edition 1984
Reprinted 1988 and 1990

Typeset by Activity Ltd, Salisbury, Wilts
Printed in Great Britain by
The University Printing House, Cambridge

British Library Cataloguing in Publication Data

Tighe, J.R.
    Pathology.-–4th ed.—(Concise medical textbooks)
    1. Pathology
    I. Title   II. Davies, D.R. (David Robert)
    III. Series
    616.07   RB111

ISBN 0-7020-0609-2

Contents

Preface

The undergraduate course in medicine becomes progressively more intensive as each specialty expands. The student is expected to read extensively in each subject yet the time available is strictly limited. This small book is intended to provide the student with a compact but readable account of histopathology covering both general and systemic pathology. It makes no pretence to being a comprehensive review but should provide the student with an introduction to the subject and facilitate revision before examinations.

Opportunity has been taken in preparing this edition for extensive revision; the chapters on general pathology have been rewritten and all the chapters on systemic pathology have had new material added. At the same time every effort has been made not to increase the size of the book.

Histopathology is largely a pictorial subject but no attempt has been made to illustrate this book, for the size would preclude a large number of illustrations and a restricted number would have limited value. Nevertheless, students are urged to see gross specimens in the post-mortem room, pathology museum and operating theatre, and to take every opportunity of studying the microscopic changes in diseased organs and tissues so that they may get a better understanding of disease processes.

A short list of books for further reading is given. Within these larger books, references to major articles are to be found and these will provide the student with a source for further reading on selected topics.

April 1984   J.R. Tighe
                                                               D.R. Davies

vii

Part I

General Pathology

1

Introduction

When a person becomes ill, the symptoms are due to a disturbance of the normal functions of some of the cells in the body. It is the business of pathology to study these disturbed functions and structural changes, to learn how they arise, how they progress and how they affect other cell systems. It also takes account of factors which restore the changes to normal. There are academic aspects and also practical considerations concerned with diagnosis and care of patients.

The first real contributions of pathology were anatomical. The work of the Italian dissectors of the 16th century showed that clinical signs and symptoms could be related to underlying lesions found at post-mortem. The subsequent use of the microscope clarified the nature of many of these lesions and led to the development of the concepts of organ and cell pathology. In the 19th and 20th centuries other techniques, notably those stemming from microbiology and biochemistry, have had an enormous impact on our concepts of disease and on the way medicine is practised.

Modern pathology is divided into subspecialties. These are histopathology (anatomical pathology), haematology, chemical pathology, microbiology and immunology. Histopathology is concerned with examination of structural changes both at post-mortem and in tissues removed from patients; cytology is a relatively new subspecialty which is concerned with the examination of isolated cells. Haematology is the study of disorders of the formed elements of the blood and of coagulation. Chemical pathology is the study of biochemical disorders, particularly as revealed by analysis of the fluids of the body. Microbiology (including virology) is the study of organisms which cause disease. Immunology is the study of phenomena associated with the specific immune response. Forensic pathology is concerned with those aspects of pathology which have legal implications.

The various subspecialties overlap and interlink, both with each other and with other medical disciplines and the basic sciences, especially in their research aspects. The absence of rigid boundaries is not surprising when it is remembered that workers in these different fields may be asking similar questions about disease processes.

When discussing causation of disease, the terms *aetiology* and *pathogenesis* are often used. Aetiological agents are those factors which play a part in causing the disease. Pathogenic mechanisms are the ways in which diseases develop. Virtually every disease has a multifactorial origin, genetic endowment and environmental influences playing their part. Even when a disease is inherited as a dominant characteristic, environmental influences may modify its expression. Some environmental agents, like trauma or some toxins, may be overwhelming in their actions, but most of them act more subtly on the individual. *Causes* may be thought of as *essential* (necessary) or *contributory* (contingent). Before Koch discovered the acid-fast bacillus, a great deal was known about the contributory causes in tuberculosis—factors such as poverty, overcrowding and malnutrition—but it is clear that tuberculosis cannot develop without the presence of the essential cause—the mycobacterium. Though it is a necessary cause, the presence of the organism is not a *sufficient* cause, for many people exposed to the organism will not develop any symptoms: the contributory causes determine how, or even if, the disease develops. There are many situations in human disease where we are in the position of knowing several contributory factors, but not an essential cause (cancer of the stomach for example), and even when we know an essential cause (as with many gene defects), we are not in a position at the moment to remedy it. It is probable that most diseases result from several factors acting together to produce the 'catastrophe' of clinical disease.

Pathological studies are used to document and elucidate the changes occurring in human disease during life and also at post-mortem. The autopsy has many different aims. There may be a medicolegal problem, in which case the aim is clear. In a clinical context it is often the 'cause of death' which is sought: this does not mean the mode of death (such as asphyxia or haemorrhage) but the essential disease process (such as carcinoma of the bronchus) which resulted in the patient's death. This has often been determined during life but it is not rare for post-mortem examination to reveal unsuspected disease. The precise cause of death is sometimes difficult to determine and occasionally one is wiser to state what the patient died 'with' rather than 'of'. Histological, chemical, microbiological, haematological and immunological techniques can all be used at post-mortem, and the information obtained employed to study the disease processes involved. The post-mortem is of greatest value when interpreted with a detailed knowledge of events and investigations during life.

The best way to understand the pathology of a disease process is to take note of many observations during its course, including those at post-mortem if death has resulted. Each of the observations may only be one frame of a film, but many frames put together give a fuller picture. It is the aim of those interested in pathology to put together the constituent frames of each disorder. With some this has been achieved in large measure but with others there are still substantial gaps. One of the attractions of pathology is its potential for filling some of the gaps.

2

Degeneration and Necrosis

When cells are deprived of oxygen or essential nutrients or when they are affected by injurious agents, they undergo functional and structural changes. Some of these changes are subtle and cannot be detected with current techniques; for example, carcinogens may cause changes in cells which may not be detectable for many years. Other forms of damage may be more easy to see; for example, damage to respiratory mechanisms, enzyme systems or membranes of the cell, can produce easily recognized changes. Sublethal damage to cells produces structural changes which are known as *degenerations*. Lethal damage to the cell causes *necrosis*.

Degeneration

The mechanisms through which injurious agents act involve interfering with one or more of the normal metabolic pathways of the cell. Oxidative respiration may be impaired by inadequate glucose or oxygen supply to the cell, as is seen in hypoglycaemia or hypoxia. Membrane functions can be impaired by heavy metals, bacterial toxins or viruses. Enzyme systems can be inhibited by free radicals. Cells can be deprived of an essential substance as a result of deficiency or competition. In general, if the abnormality is more than very transitory, structural changes appear. Some of these effects can be seen by naked-eye examination, others require conventional light microscopy, but some need electron microscopy or other techniques. Some biochemical lesions occur without detectable morphological changes.

Intracellular oedema occurs when hypoxia, infection or poisons damage the 'sodium pump' and water accumulates inside cells. The affected tissues appear swollen and paler than normal; the edge of the cut surface of affected organs tends to bulge over the capsule. Microscopically the boundaries of the swollen cell become less distinct and the cytoplasm more opaque than normal (sometimes called 'cloudy swelling'); later, vacuoles appear ('vacuolar degeneration') and when it becomes severe the whole cytoplasm becomes very pale and homogeneous ('hydropic degeneration'). These changes are seen after many insults.

Fat exists in the body mainly in the form of neutral fat in adipose tissue cells and as lipoproteins in other cells and plasma. *Fatty change* is the

5

accumulation of stainable neutral fat in parenchymal cells. The term does not refer to collections of true fat cells in tissue, which is called *adiposity*. Fatty change can be seen on naked-eye examination in, for example, the heart muscle in chronic severe anaemia, where it gives yellowish streaks in the otherwise dark muscle. Similarly, a chronic alcoholic may have a pale enlarged liver which is greasy to the touch. In conventional microscopic slides the fat, which dissolves out in processing, is represented by large empty spaces within the cells; the fat can be stained in frozen sections, which do not pass through fat solvents. The fat in liver parenchymal cells is not derived from the breakdown of lipoprotein within the cell but from fatty acids which arrive in the bloodstream. Normally the liver cells use these fatty acids, with amino acids, to make lipoproteins. If this metabolic pathway is impaired, neutral fat accumulates. Probably the commonest cause of hepatic fatty change in Britain is alcohol. Protein deprivation, particularly of the lipotropic factors choline and methionine, also causes this change, and a very severe version of this is seen in kwashiorkor in children in the Tropics.

Another form of fatty change is seen in the degenerative vascular disease atheroma. Accumulation of lipid-laden cells in the intima of larger arteries is an early change in this disorder, which can ultimately cause occlusion of the vessel.

Hyaline is a widely used word in pathology but it is purely descriptive, referring to a histological appearance, and has no biochemical specificity. It originally meant glass-like but is now loosely used and in general refers to a microscopic appearance of an abnormal homogeneous area, usually staining with eosin, sometimes in the cytoplasm of cells, but it can also refer to extracellular changes. It is a convenient term for indicating an abnormality but does not convey its precise nature. An example of intracellular hyaline is Mallory's hyaline, an area of cytoplasmic degeneration seen in liver cells of patients with alcoholic hepatitis. Hyaline droplets in the proximal convoluted tubule of the kidney occur when there is heavy protein loss through the glomeruli and subsequent resorption through the tubule. Several forms of focal cytoplasmic degeneration, with different electron microscopical specificities, are seen by light microscopy as 'hyaline'.

Abnormal accumulations within cells

Congenital enzyme deficiencies may lead to abnormal accumulations of substances within cells. Glycogen storage disease, of which there are seven types, is a form affecting carbohydrate metabolism. The best known is von Gierke's disease in which there is a deficiency of glucose-6-phosphatase, which is necessary for the conversion of glucose-6-phosphate to glucose. The resultant excess of glucose-6-phosphate leads to massive accumulations of glycogen in liver and kidneys. McArdle's syndrome and Pompe's disease are two other forms of glycogen storage disease in which skeletal and cardiac muscle are infiltrated.

Other storage diseases result from inherited deficiencies of *lysosomal enzymes* which lead to accumulation of lipid within the cells. Gaucher's disease is an example in which glucosidase is deficient and ceramide glucoside accumulates in histiocytes in the lymphohistiocytic system, giving rise to splenomegaly and hepatomegaly. Similarly, sphingomyelinase deficiency leads to sphingomyelin accumulation (Niemann–Pick disease), and hexosaminidase A deficiency gives a ganglioside accumulation (Tay–Sachs disease). These are rare conditions but give rise to striking clinical and pathological appearances.

Necrosis

Necrosis is usually defined as the death of a cell or cells in continuity with living tissue. It is distinguished from autolysis (which is the post-mortem change that occurs when the whole organism dies) but has some features in common. At the edge of a necrotic lesion a reaction of the living to the dead tissue develops and this modifies appearances. Very early necrotic lesions are difficult to see with conventional histology but may be demonstrated by histochemistry. Cell death results from an interruption of one of the processes which maintain its life and there are very many causes. Perhaps the commonest necrotic lesions encountered clinically are those which result from the obstruction of the lumen of an artery, such as myocardial and cerebral infarcts. Infections also cause necrosis—pus is partly composed of dead cells. Other causes of necrosis include chemicals (e.g. mercury causing necrosis of renal tubular cells), radiation and immunological reactions. Some cells are more susceptible to damage than others. Cerebral neurons survive only for about 4 minutes after interruption of their blood supply (which is why procedures to restart the heart must be instituted immediately after cardiac arrest if they are to be effective). On the other hand, skeletal muscle fibres can survive interruption of their blood supply for a considerably longer time without suffering irreversible damage.

Necrotic tissue may remain of firm consistency (*coagulative necrosis*) or may liquefy (*colliquative necrosis*). This latter change is seen particularly in the central nervous system. *Caseation* is a form of coagulative necrosis which has a cream cheese-like appearance on naked-eye examination; it is particularly seen in tuberculosis. *Gangrene* is necrosis with putrefaction, that is with growth of saprophytic organisms in the dead tissue ('wet gangrene'). The term gangrene is also applied to infarction at the extremities of a limb following ischaemia—when infarction is followed by desiccation and discoloration without putrefaction ('dry gangrene').

Under the microscope the commonest changes seen in the cell in necrosis are swelling of the cytoplasm (due to an increased content of water) and the break-up of the nucleus. The nucleus may fade away (*karyolysis*) or may lose its normal chromatin pattern and become small and more darkly stained (*pyknosis*) and then it fragments and disperses (*karyorrhexis*). At the junction of dead and viable tissue the processes of inflammation and healing may be seen. Removal of dead tissue and its replacement by specialized cells or fibrous tissue occurs if the effects of the injurious agent are contained. An important change in necrotic cells is the release of intracellular enzymes into the interstitium and thence into the circulation. These enzymes can be detected in the serum and are diagnostically useful.

Apoptosis is a process of individual cell death and disposal which occurs physiologically (in cell turnover in organs such as the liver) and also pathologically in conditions such as atrophy. It is observed microscopically, no necrotic lesion being visible on naked-eye examination. Other patterns of single-cell necrosis are also seen in pathology; it is often seen in viral infections, for example infectious hepatitis has many small foci of dead liver cells, accompanied by inflammation, scattered through the hepatic lobules. In severe cases the necrotic cells may become confluent to give larger lesions.

'Degenerative' changes in connective tissue

In disease there are a number of non-specific changes occurring in connective tissue which are frequently referred to as degenerative. This is not an ideal word, for often the change is due to production of new tissue or matrix in situ, or to the accumulation of proteins from the bloodstream. The term is used widely, however, sometimes as a cloak for ignorance, sometimes as a convenient shorthand.

Fibrinoid change

This simply means that an area stains like fibrin. The abnormality is usually seen in the walls of blood vessels or in collagenous connective tissue, sometimes accompanied by an inflammatory reaction. In some cases it really is due to fibrin being present, as in the walls of small blood vessels in accelerated hypertension. In other situations immunoglobulins may be the predominant protein, as in some deposits in rheumatoid arthritis. (The nature of the deposit is identified by immunohistochemistry.) Because fibrinoid change is often due to proteins leaking into an area from the bloodstream, the term *insudation* is used in this context. Also cell death sometimes accompanies the process, in which case *fibrinoid necrosis* is the term used.

Hyaline change

As with cellular hyaline, this is a purely descriptive term. It refers to the pale eosinophilic, amorphous hypocellular appearance seen particularly in collagenous connective tissue and sometimes smooth muscle. Again there is no biochemical specificity. One of the commonest examples is hyaline arteriolar sclerosis seen in ageing, hypertension and diabetes mellitus; this change in the vessel wall is in part due to an accumulation of glycoproteins derived from the bloodstream and in part to increased cross-linkage of collagen fibrils. Scar tissue becomes hyalinized as it matures. Leiomyomas in the uterus sometimes undergo very extensive hyalinization of the collagen within them.

Mucoid (myxoid) change

An increased amount of glycosaminoglycans is often seen in connective tissue subject to chronic low-grade trauma. In haematoxylin and eosin sections this appears as pools of loose, slightly basophilic connective tissue. Such an appearance is seen in the development of cystic ganglia close to joints. Excessive accumulations also occur in the media of the aorta in cystic medial degeneration. In the genetic defects of glycosaminoglycan metabolism (the mucopolysaccharidoses), there are accumulations of these substances in many tissues. A similar change may result from some epithelial tumours, e.g. breast cancer, producing vast excess of mucin.

Elastotic change

Collagenous connective tissue sometimes acquires the staining characteristics of elastic tissue. The commonest example of this is seen in skin subject to prolonged exposure to u.v. light, when the collagen of the dermis develops marked elastotic changes (often called solar damage because of its association with sunlight).

Dystrophic calcification

Following tissue damage, calcification sometimes occurs, for example when thyroid nodules degenerate, when large atheromatous plaques develop in arteries, or in the fibrous scars of old tuberculosis. This calcification occurs with a normal serum level of calcium.

Calcification occurs in otherwise normal tissue when the serum calcium is raised. This is often called *metastatic calcification* and is particularly seen in hyperparathyroidism and vitamin D overdose.

Amyloid

This is rather different from the other changes discussed here. Amyloid was originally recognized as an abnormal material laid down in connective tissue and, because it stained with iodine and acid, was called amyloid ('like starch'). It is quite unlike starch in other ways and has been shown to consist of a group of fibrillary proteins which have in common an antiparallel β-plicated sheet structure. This physical characteristic gives the amyloids their staining characteristics, the most useful of which is the green birefringence when stained with Congo red. Deposits of amyloid lead to atrophy of parenchymal cells, to ischaemia because of vessel narrowing, and to functional effects such as proteinuria. Early studies showed that there are a wide range of clinical effects but that cases fell into three patterns. *Primary* amyloid occurred without obvious precipitating cause. It particularly involved heart, skin, tongue, and alimentary and respiratory tracts. *Secondary* amyloid was associated with chronic inflammatory diseases such as tuberculosis and rheumatoid arthritis; it particularly affected liver, spleen, adrenals and kidney. *Localized* amyloid occurred as small deposits, often in the elderly, usually with little functional significance. Advances in diagnostic methods led to erosion of the primary group, especially when it was discovered that many cases were associated with plasma cell and lymphoid dyscrasias. Molecular chemistry has shown that there are two major amyloid proteins, AA (related to the protein SAA in the serum) and AL (related to light chains of immunoglobulins) as well as some rarer forms.

The most useful current classification of amyloid is as follows.

1. Systemic
    i. Associated with immune dyscrasias, especially multiple myeloma (AL).
    ii. Associated with chronic inflammation (AA).
    iii. Heredofamilial forms (AA in familial Mediterranean fever).
2. Organ limited and localized, including endocrine-gland-associated amyloid (medullary carcinoma of the thyroid and islets of Langerhans) and senile amyloid (small plaques found in several organs in the elderly).

The systemic versions are serious progressive diseases leading to death in those afflicted. In the second group the amyloid is only occasionally responsible for clinical disease.

3

Inflammation and Healing

The body's defences against injurious agents include non-specific defences such as (1) an intact epithelium, (2) secretions from the epithelium, for example lysozyme in tears or acid in gastric juice, (3) bronchial ciliary action, the cough reflex and the sneeze reflex which prevent foreign material reaching the lung via the air passages, (4) the acute inflammatory reaction, (5) non-specific phagocytosis by histiocytes, (6) bactericidal tissue fluids, and (7) certain metabolic differences which make some organisms able to damage cells of one species, but not of another. There are also specific defence mechanisms which act against recognized foreign antigens and, properly directed, lead to their elimination without damage to the host. This latter group is described as being part of the specific immune response (see Chapter 4).

Inflammation is loosely described as the response of the body to injury. This implies an active response, both local and generalized, extending beyond the cells which are injured. Injurious agents are the same as those causing cell degeneration and necrosis and include organisms (especially bacteria but also viruses, fungi, protozoa, parasites), chemicals, physical agents (radiation, heat, cold, electricity, mechanical trauma), hypersensitivity and ischaemia. Bacterial infection provides good examples of inflammatory processes and these are taken as a model. Some cell damage, e.g. that which results in neoplastic change, does not result in inflammation.

There are two main patterns of inflammatory processes—acute and chronic. These words were originally applied to a timescale but have come to imply a pattern of cellular reaction. A more precise definition of acute inflammation is the reaction of vascular and supporting elements of a tissue to injury, resulting in the formation of an exudate, provided the injury has not been so severe as to destroy the area. Chronic inflammatory processes are those in which destruction and inflammation are taking place at the same time as attempts at healing. Variations on these two patterns occur and terms such as 'subacute' and 'acute on chronic' may be encountered.

The acute inflammatory reaction

A very good clinical example of an acute inflammatory reaction is a boil

11

in the skin. This is an infection caused by an organism (often a staphylococcus) entering through a break in the epithelium and multiplying beneath it. It shows the 'cardinal signs' of inflammation, which are *calor, dolor, rubor, tumor* (heat, pain, redness, swelling), together with impairment of function. Often there is a rapid onset and a successful outcome involves localization of the organisms and their removal, with the tissue restored to normal. However, the result of an acute inflammatory reaction depends on a balance of host and agent factors. Possible results of infection of the skin with staphylococci include the following.

1. *Resolution*—complete return of injured tissue to normal. This is the most desirable result and often occurs when tissue destruction has not been too great.

2. *Suppuration*—the formation of pus, composed of polymorphonuclear leucocytes together with partly liquefied dead tissue. If the pus is localized within the tissues, an abscess forms. If an epithelial surface breaks down over the pus, then an *ulcer* is formed.

3. *Spread* of the infection may occur. Instead of becoming localized an infection may spread directly through soft tissues. This process is known as *cellulitis*. Sometimes pus will track along a narrow tissue plane opening out onto the surface. This blind-ended track is then called a *sinus*. If the track connects two epithelial surfaces, it is known as a *fistula*. When pus forms in the pleural cavity it often spreads between the visceral and parietal pleura and is known as *empyema*. Organisms may enter lymphatics and spread along these giving *lymphangitis*, and then reach the draining lymph nodes where inflammation is known as *lymphadenitis*. When this occurs there is usually a red mark from the site of the original infection to the lymph node showing the path of the inflamed lymphatic. Spread via the bloodstream may also occur. The presence of organisms in the blood is termed *bacteraemia*. Normally the organisms are quickly removed by the process of phagocytosis, but sometimes they increase in numbers in the blood and the patient becomes seriously ill, the diseased state being called *septicaemia*. If particles of pus containing pyogenic micro-organisms are carried in the bloodstream and settle in the tissues to produce widespread abscesses, a state of *pyaemia* is said to have developed. When acute infection reaches and involves serous membranes, a fluid exudate often forms—*ascites*, or *pleural* and *pericardial effusions*. The exudate may be clear (*serous*) but it is more likely to contain pus (*purulent*) or consist mainly of fibrin (a *fibrinous exudate*). Another membrane which may become involved in acute inflammation is the pia-arachnoid of the meninges, in which case an acute meningitis results.

4. *Chronic inflammation.* If the host is unable to eliminate the organism and the presence of the organism does not result in the immediate death of the host, then the pattern of inflammation changes from acute to chronic.

5. *Fibrosis*. When tissue disruption has been too great for resolution to occur, scarring may be the end-result when the organism is eliminated.

6. *Death* occurs when the host is unable to contain the effects of the organism. Such an outcome was not rare in the pre-antibiotic era, when relatively minor infections spread and resulted in death from septicaemia. Infection is still the mode of death nowadays for many patients debilated by other diseases.

Development

The development of the acute inflammatory reaction has been extensively studied in man and experimental animals. The two major events are the *vascular response* and the *formation of an exudate*. Shortly after tissue injury there is a change in the calibre of blood vessels and also in the characteristics of the vessel wall. There is an initial constriction of vessels which is transient and soon followed by the more important vasodilatation. This dilatation is partly controlled by an axon reflex but nevertheless occurs in the absence of a nerve supply as a result of locally released chemical mediators. Following the change in calibre there is also an initial increased flow through the capillaries, soon to be followed by stasis of blood within the capillaries. The endothelial cells tend to swell and the polymorphonuclear leucocytes stick to them and ultimately emigrate into the interstitial space. Formation of the exudate is the second major component of the acute inflammatory reaction and increased capillary permeability is essential for this. The exudate is formed of fluid and cells from the bloodstream. The fluid is protein rich. The cellular exudate is mainly composed of polymorphonuclear leucocytes which emigrate through the capillary wall by active amoeboid movement influenced by chemotactic substances in the injured area. Red blood cells may also appear in the exudate but they are simply carried out passively with the plasma (a process called *diapedesis*). The acute inflammatory reaction provides a mechanism for the rapid deployment of the phagocytic neutrophil polymorphonuclear leucocytes to the area.

The outcome of an acute inflammatory reaction is determined by host factors and factors peculiar to the organism. Host factors include such things as the blood supply to the area, the competence of the polymorphonuclear leucocytes and other phagocytic cells, the immune state and the age of the individual. Factors to do with the organism would include the size of dose (a small number of bacteria being more easily dealt with than a large number of bacteria), and route of administration (many bacteria ingested into the stomach would be killed by the acid juice, whereas the same organisms entering a breach in the skin might cause a severe infection). Substances produced by the organism influence the pattern of the infection. Exotoxins are substances which diffuse out from the organism. *Staphylococcus aureus* produces an exotoxin called coagulase which converts fibrinogen to fibrin and tends to wall off the infection to produce an abscess. On the other hand, *Streptococcus pyogenes* produces hyaluronidase and other substances which break down tissue components and cause the spread of the organisms through the tissue giving a cellulitis. Some organisms produce toxins that are absorbed and have effects elsewhere in the body, for example infection with *Clostridium tetani* shows little local reaction but death results from the action of the toxin on the nervous system. Breakdown of bacterial cell walls and release of endotoxin can produce a state of shock which has a profound influence on the outcome of infection. The antigenicity of an organism may play a part in the ultimate outcome of an infection but has little to do with the initial events of an infection, unless it is in a previously exposed individual, when immune mechanisms may prevent any tissue damage.

If tissue damage is small and the injurious agent is removed, then the polymorphs are soon replaced by histiocytes (mononuclear phagocytes) which mop up damaged tissue in this *demolition* phase and resolution occurs. The acute inflammatory reaction is part of the body's non-specific defences. Specific immunological factors may modify the course but are not an essential part of the reaction.

At this stage it is easy to understand how the cardinal signs of inflammation come about. The warmth (*calor*) is due to increased blood flow, whereas the increased amount of blood within vessels in the tissue gives the redness (*rubor*) of the area. The swelling (*tumor*) is due to the formation of exudate, the pain (*dolor*) due to stimulation of pain receptors by tissue damage and increased tension within the tissue. The amount of loss of function depends on the extent of the inflammation and which site is involved. A localized acute inflammatory reaction often has *systemic effects* if it is severe enough. The most prominent are often a rise in temperature (pyrexia), a rise in number of neutrophil polymorphonuclear leucocytes in the bloodstream (a neutrophil leucocytosis) and a quickening of the pulse. These are due to chemical mediators returning from the site to the systemic circulation.

Chemical control

The factors which control the vascular response and formation of the exudate are largely chemical, though neural factors can influence them. Many chemical mediators affect the acute inflammatory process. *Amines* have been identified as playing a part since the role of histamine was shown in the pathogenesis of *the triple response* (the red line, flare and wheal which follow stroking of the skin). *Kinins* are substances which cause contraction of smooth muscle, and one of these—bradykinin—causes vasodilatation, increased vascular permeability and pain. Also in the plasma there are kinin-forming enzymes such as kallikrein and plasmin which cause the conversion of kininogen to bradykinin. When complement is activated, factors are released which are chemotactic for leucocytes. The complement system, the coagulation system and the fibrinolytic system are all interrelated and involved in inflammation. When *polymorphonuclear leucocytes* are damaged they release a number of proteases and other proteins which increase vascular permeability. *Platelets*, which may be activated by tissue injury, contain *serotonin* (5-HT) and *prostaglandins*, both of which increase vascular permeability. The *leukotrienes* (molecules closely related to prostaglandin) have been shown to be responsible for the activity attributed to slow-reacting substance (SRS) in the earlier literature and cause sustained increase in permeability lasting for hours.

The mediators have especially important roles in bringing about *capillary dilatation, increasing capillary permeability* and in *influencing the behaviour of inflammatory cells*. The interrelationships of these and other chemical mediators are complex and are different in various pathological conditions. The outcome of an acute inflammatory reaction caused by an infection or other injurious stimulus is determined by a balance of host factors and factors peculiar to the injurious stimulus.

The cells of inflammatory reactions

Neutrophil polymorphonuclear leucocytes are produced in the bone marrow, circulate in the bloodstream and are rapidly deployed in acute inflammatory reactions. They have multilobed nuclei and their cytoplasm contains both neutrophil granules (which contain lysozyme and lactoferrin) and azurophil granules (which contain bactericidal enzymes such as neutral proteases, myeloperoxidase, lysozyme and acid hydrolases). The granules are not distinct in histological slides, and haematological preparations show them best. A major function of these cells is phagocytosis, a process which, for some substances, is assisted by the presence of receptors for complement (C3$_b$ fraction) and immunoglobulin (Fc portion) on the neutrophil surface. Digestion of phagocytosed material occurs within the cells, but neutrophils can also release their active chemicals into the tissues. When people talk of 'acute inflammatory cells' or 'pus cells', these are the cells which are implied.

Eosinophils are also produced in the bone marrow and circulate in the bloodstream. They have bilobed nuclei and eosinophilic cytoplasmic granules. The function of these cells remains unclear, though they are frequently seen in parasitic infections and type I hypersensitivity reactions. It seems likely that they may modify basophil reactions and have an anti-parasitic function.

Mast cells are mainly found in the tissue; they are very similar to the basophils that are occasionally seen in the bloodstream but are believed to be a different population. They are especially numerous in mucous membranes and in connective tissue. The cytoplasm of these cells contains many potent chemicals which when released act as mediators of inflammation. They include histamine, slow-reacting substance of anaphylaxis (leukotriene), eosinophil chemotactic factor of anaphylaxis and platelet-activating factor which causes platelets to undergo a release reaction. The granules are released following several stimuli including type I hypersensitivity reactions (p. 30).

Lymphocytes are usually seen in tissue sections as small round cells with a dense nucleus and not very much cytoplasm. When stimulated, however, they can become larger cells with more open nuclei and more abundant cytoplasm, and may be difficult to distinguish from histiocytes. The two major functional types are the B lymphocytes, which become plasma cells and produce immunoglobulin, and the T lymphocytes, which are responsible for cell-mediated reactions, partly via the production of lymphokines (see Chapter 4). Lymphocytes, plasma cells and histiocytes are often collectively called 'chronic inflammatory cells'.

Plasma cells are round or oval cells, each with an eccentric nucleus showing coarsely clumped chromatin. The cytoplasm is amphophilic and can be shown to be filled with immunoglobulin which is secreted by the cell. They are formed from B lymphocytes.

Histiocytes, when actively phagocytic, are also called macrophages. They are found in the tissues; in the bloodstream they are called monocytes. This is the other group of 'professional phagocytes' which, with the neutrophil polymorphonuclear leucocytes, have a well-developed phagocytic capacity for the removal of foreign agents and damaged cells. The neutrophils are equipped for quick deployment and rapid function, but the histiocytes are much longer lived and mount a more sustained reaction. Though part of the 'non-specific defences', they can be recruited by lymphocytes to take part in specific immune reactions.

Under normal circumstances, histiocytes have rounded or kidney-shaped nuclei with open chromatin and plentiful, slightly foamy cytoplasm. In some situations the cytoplasm becomes more abundant and eosinophilic so that they resemble squamous epithelial cells and are called *epithelioid cells*. It seems that this occurs when the histiocytes develop secretory organelles in the cytoplasm. Under some circumstances, usually when they cannot properly deal with material to be phagocytosed, histiocytes fuse and become *multinucleate giant cells*. These can be seen in different forms: *foreign body* giant cells tend to have the nuclei clumped together in the centre of the cell; the *Langhans type* giant cell (seen in tuberculosis and other immune granulomas) has the nuclei arranged around the periphery of the cell like a horseshoe. A circumscribed collection of histiocytes, with or without giant cells, constitutes a *granuloma*.

Healing

In pathology, 'healing' means the replacement of dead or damaged tissue by new viable tissue. If the replacement is by specialized cells similar to those lost, the process is called *regeneration*. If the replacement is by fibrous tissue, it is called *repair*. Regenerative capacity varies considerably between cell lines. Cells with a rapid turnover under normal circumstances are called *labile cells* and in general have a good regenerative capacity, e.g. many epithelial cells, bone marrow and lymph node cells. A healthy person can be a blood or marrow donor and quickly replace the lost cells. At the other extreme, the *permanent cells* (or post-mitotic cells) are incapable of mitosis and when destroyed must be replaced by fibrosis (or gliosis, in the case of the central nervous system). The myocardial fibres which die after a heart attack cannot be regenerated and the dead area is replaced by a fibrous scar. Neurons are also cells which do not regenerate (axon regrowth occurs but this requires a viable cell body and a nerve sheath). Between these two extremes are the *stable cells* which are capable of mitosis but have a slower turnover than the labile cells. These vary in their regenerative capacity, for example liver parenchymal cells regenerate easily but cartilage is poorly replaced. Despite a great deal of research, the controls affecting regenerating cells remain obscure.

The healing of surgical incisions provides good examples of the processes involved. Two patterns are conventionally described: healing by first or second intention. These are ends of a spectrum rather than distinct processes.

Healing by *first intention* is the pattern seen with a clean, incised surgical wound with minimum destruction of tissue, the edges of the wound being closely opposed and healing occurring without complication. There is an initial small *haematoma* with a mild acute inflammatory reaction alongside the damaged tissue but the exudate remains small. *Epithelial proliferation* occurs and quickly (within 24 hours) seals across the wound at the level of the basal cells of the epidermis. It separates a superficial scab of haematoma and exudate from the dermal and subcutaneous wound. As epithelial proliferation continues, the scab is pushed more superficially and is ultimately shed. *Histiocytes* of the demolition phase of the acute inflammatory reaction remove the small amount of damaged tissue deeper in the wound. By about the third day, *capillaries* have sprouted into the damaged area and with them are fibroblasts and histiocytes, this tissue being known as *granulation tissue* (because of its granular appearance when seen at the base of a large open wound). Granulation tissue is an extremely important element in the healing of many damaged tissues. The fibroblasts form collagen and after about seven days there is a firm bond. As well as their secretory function, the *fibroblasts* also have a contractile function and many of them develop a prominent actin content in their cytoplasm (when they are called *myofibroblasts*). These cells serve to contract down the immature connective tissue and help to ensure a small scar. The end-result is an intact epithelium (regeneration) and a small fibrous scar (repair)—the most satisfactory result following surgery.

There are some differences when the wound is large, when the edges cannot be brought together or when complications such as infection occur. In these situations sealing of epithelium across the wound does not occur early, there is more granulation tissue and the end-result is more tissue distortion and a large scar. This pattern of wound healing is often called healing by *second intention* and is exemplified by the healing of a large wound with widely separated edges. Initial events are similar but the haematoma is larger and there is more inflammation because of greater tissue destruction. Epithelial proliferation again begins at an early stage but cannot immediately bridge the wound, and hence has to grow down and spread progressively across it, at the junction of viable tissue and exudate. Concurrently the demolition phase of the acute inflammatory reaction removes damaged tissue in the base of the wound, and capillaries with accompanying fibroblasts and histiocytes sprout into the wound from the subcutaneous tissue. The ingrowth of capillaries into exudate and dead tissue is called 'organization'. This granulation tissue is even more important in second intention healing for the contraction of the wound, brought about by the myofibroblasts and starting at about the second day, results in considerable diminution in the size of the wound and hence in the amount of new tissue which has to be formed. Ultimately the epithelium grows right across the wound (regeneration) and a comparatively large scar forms (repair). It is interesting that the more specialized parts of the skin—the hair follicles and sweat glands—do not regenerate.

In surgical practice many *complications* of wound healing may be seen. It is convenient to group them as early and late complications. In general the early ones are the result of infection, which is commoner in large open wounds than in those that heal by first intention. But infection occurring in a small wound has the effect of producing more tissue destruction and results in the pattern of healing by second intention. Infection with pyogenic organisms can lead to *abscess*, *sinus* or *fistula* formation. An abscess may develop around a suture (*stitch abscess*). *Cellulitis* can occur, spreading out from the edges of the wound. *Dehiscence* (complete breakdown of the wound) sometimes occurs, especially with large abdominal incisions with an underlying peritonitis. When there is dead tissue remaining in a wound and spores of an anaerobic organism are introduced (not a common event in well-regulated practice), serious complications like *gas gangrene* (*Clostridium welchii*) or tetanus (*Clostridium tetani*) may follow.

The late complications tend to be abnormalities of fibrous tissue formation. *Stretching* may result if there is excessive tension on the wound; if this occurs, a *hernia* may develop. Scar tissue can proliferate excessively to form tumour-like masses (*keloid scars*) which are commoner around the head and neck and in blacks. *Cicatrization* is an excessive contraction of a scar occurring late and producing tissue distortion. Proliferation of Schwann cells and axons on the cut end of a nerve can produce a little nodule known as an *amputation neuroma*; this can be painful, especially if caught up in scar tissue. Squamous epithelium introduced deep into the wound area at the time of operation can form a small cyst: the epithelium continues to grow and the cyst lumen fills with keratin—this is an *epidermoid cyst* which may present late. These little nodules have to be distinguished from tumour deposits which can recur in a scar following an operation for cancer.

Most surgical wounds heal with no problem but there are local and systemic factors which impair healing. At the site it is important that infection, dead tissue and foreign material are eliminated before full healing occurs. (By 'foreign material' is meant substances which are recognized by the body as foreign, for good healing occurs in the presence of inert foreign substances such as some sutures and prostheses.) An inadequate blood supply produces ischaemia and delays healing. Excessive mobility prevents neat scar formation; so also does tethering of the skin to an underlying structure (like the anterior surface of the tibia) which prevents good apposition of wound margins. If an incision passes through residual malignant tumour, then complete healing is unlikely.

Systemic factors which impair healing include nutritional deficiencies (protein, vitamin C, zinc) and hormonal state (high levels of glucocorticoids). Elderly people also seem to have delayed healing compared with the young.

Fracture healing

The end-result of uncomplicated fracture healing is bone which is indistinguishable from normal. When a bone has been fractured and the two broken ends are in alignment, the intervening space is first filled with blood clot (a haematoma). This is quickly invaded by fibroblasts extending from the periosteum of the broken ends of bone, followed by osteoblasts which lay down the protein matrix of bone, called osteoid (collagen plus glycosaminoglycans), in which the broken ends become embedded. The dead fragments of bone adjacent to the fracture are reabsorbed by osteoclasts. The new osteoid becomes calcified but it is more irregular and bulky than normal bone. Its collagen fibres are irregularly arranged and it is therefore called 'woven bone'; it is this which forms the temporary bony union called callus. This is gradually remodelled by osteoclastic and osteoblastic cells to mature lamellar bone. The precise factors controlling the return to normal are not clear but stress on the bone plays its part.

Chronic inflammation

Chronic inflammatory diseases are those which continue for a long time (weeks at least) and in which inflammation and cell damage are present at the same time as healing processes. There are many causes and many different features, but in general these disorders can be grouped into 1) those which result from *failure of resolution* of an acute inflammatory reaction, and 2) those which have a very *inconspicuous acute phase*. In both groups the cellular infiltrate is usually composed mainly of chronic inflammatory cells (lymphocytes, plasma cells and histiocytes) whether or not other cells are present. The picture is much more variable and certainly not as stereotyped as the early phase of acute inflammation. Often the effect and mechanisms of the specific response dominate the picture.

Failure of resolution

When an acute inflammatory reaction fails to eliminate an injurious agent, cell damage proceeds but healing processes will also be initiated. Granulation tissue is formed, fibrous tissue develops and regeneration may begin: the cellular infiltrate changes from being predominantly polymorphonuclear to being predominantly chronic inflammatory cell in type. Polymorphs are often present in the active centres of cell damage. A picture like this is seen in the development of a chronic abscess following failure of resolution of acute suppurative inflammation. Infection with a pyogenic organism produces tissue death and an infiltrate of polymorphs, many of which are also killed, giving rise to thick, yellowish, semifluid pus. A small amount of pus may be resolved but a large amount either has to discharge to a surface or become localized. If it becomes localized, it is surrounded by a wall (the 'pyogenic membrane') of granulation tissue outside which fibrous tissue develops. The wall has polymorphs on the inside but in the later stages there are many chronic inflammatory cells in the outer layers. Resolution then becomes difficult, though the contents may become sterile. Fortunately chronic abscesses are now much less common than in the pre-antibiotic era.

Inconspicuous acute phase

In those chronic inflammatory processes with an inconspicuous acute phase, one group (I) is characterized by the presence of histiocytic granulomas. The second group (II) is a miscellaneous mixture of chronic inflammatory diseases.

Group I

A *granuloma* is a circumscribed collection of histiocytes, often with multinucleate forms and sometimes showing central necrosis. Though the words are similar, a histiocytic granuloma is quite a different thing from granulation tissue and the two should not be confused. Unfortunately the term granuloma is sometimes used very loosely to indicate almost any chronic inflammatory process.

Foreign body granulomas occur in connective tissue around insoluble material which the histiocytes cannot phagocytose. A good example is that which is sometimes seen around a stitch left in the tissue. Histiocytes gather around the foreign material and some of them become multinucleate foreign body giant cells by fusion. Typically these have the nuclei crowded together in the centre of the giant cell. Small fragments of the material may be phagocytosed by histiocytes but large pieces are not engulfed. This type of reaction is part of the non-specific phagocytic function of histiocytes. It does not require the material to be antigenic. It does, however, require it to have certain surface characteristics for some foreign materials do not elicit this response. Some materials which are not truly foreign to the body, but which find themselves in an abnormal position, also provoke this reaction, e.g. hair in a pilonidal sinus, cholesterol in the gall-bladder wall, keratin from a ruptured epidermoid cyst.

Immune granulomas are seen in some chronic infections (such as tuberculosis) and in some similar diseases where an infectious agent has not been identified (e.g. sarcoidosis, Crohn's disease). They are also seen in a few diseases in which disordered immunity occurs (e.g. primary biliary cirrhosis). There is evidence that many of these granulomas form as a result of substances produced by T lymphocytes (lymphokines) which concentrate histiocytes in one area.

Tuberculosis is caused by an acid-fast bacillus. *Mycobacterium tuberculosis* is responsible for most cases in Britain, though *M. bovis* also causes human disease in other countries. These organisms cause little initial damage and have evolved the capacity to evade the non-specific defence mechanisms and to live in histiocytes. The two main forms of the disease are childhood (also called primary) and adult (secondary). In childhood pulmonary TB an air-borne infection results in a small sub-pleural inflammatory reaction (the Ghon focus), mainly in the mid-zone of the lung. The draining lymph nodes in the mediastinum become enlarged, sometimes considerably. The combination of a focus and lymph nodes is known as the Ghon complex. The histology of the focus is believed to be an initial transient mild acute inflammatory reaction, the lesion being quickly infiltrated by histiocytes and lymphocytes. Acid-fast bacilli are phagocytosed by histiocytes. Some of the histiocytes develop plentiful eosinophilic cytoplasm and resemble squamous epithelial cells. These are called epithelioid cells and are frequently seen in this sort of granuloma; they represent a change in the cytoplasmic organelles of the histiocytes. Some of the histiocytes fuse to form multinucleate giant cells which often have the nuclei arranged around the periphery in a horseshoe pattern (Langhans type giant cells). If the granuloma enlarges, it may undergo central necrosis. In a community where tuberculosis is common many children develop such lesions but most of them heal provided that the child is well nourished and has a competent immune system. It seems that stimulation of a T lymphocyte response results in the histiocytes being able to kill the acid-fast bacilli growing inside them. The result would be a small scar in the lung and possibly a calcified lymph node.

In some children, however, the bacilli overcome the host defences and the disease spreads. It can do this locally: as the Ghon focus is subpleural, pleural involvement easily occurs and effusions arise in the pleural cavity. If the focus enlarges and involves a bronchus, then infected material can enter the bronchus and can either be expectorated or distributed around the bronchial tree producing bronchopneumonia. If a blood vessel is invaded, then vascular spread around the body sets up foci of infection in many organs and in each focus new granulomas develop. This very serious complication may be seen at autopsy, with the multiple small deposits being likened to millet seeds: the term miliary tuberculosis is still applied to this picture.

In adult tuberculosis the picture is rather different. It used to be believed that the differences were due to previous exposure to tuberculosis, but it is probable that the adult reacts in a different way from the child, even if not previously exposed. If we again consider the pulmonary version of the disease, the major lesion is usually found at the apex of one of the upper lobes (an Assman focus). It is usually larger than the Ghon focus and the granulomas are more likely to undergo extensive central necrosis, giving a softening. (When such a lesion is seen with the naked eye the necrosis has an appearance rather like cream cheese— hence the term caseation.) These lesions are likely to track to a bronchus and discharge leaving a cavitating lesion at the apex. This may then heal, with fibrosis and sometimes calcification. Caseation and fibrosis are usually more marked in the adult-type disease, and lymph node enlargement is not as prominent as in the childhood pattern. The infected material which reaches the bronchus may be coughed up but, especially in elderly and debilitated patients, it may be distributed around the bronchial tree and produce tuberculous bronchopneumonia. Direct spread occurs to pleura and adjacent lung, lymphatic spread gives rise to lymphadenopathy, and miliary spread can also occur. In the late stages coughed-up bacilli are swallowed and lesions occur along the gastrointestinal tract.

Adult-type tuberculosis also occurs in bone, in the kidney and lower genitourinary tract, in the alimentary tract and sometimes in other organs.

Leprosy is another infection caused by acid-fast bacilli (*Mycobacterium leprae*). There are said to be more than 11×10^6 cases in the world, mainly in the Tropics. Spread of infection is on a person-to-person basis and many infections heal completely without symptoms. It usually takes about three years after infection for clinical manifestations to appear, for it is a slow-growing organism. The disease is very interesting from the point of view of the mechanisms involved, for there is a spectrum of clinical manifestations paralleled by histological changes which reflect the state of competence of the individual's cell-mediated immune reactions. These histological changes vary from tuberculoid granulomas (tuberculoid) to a diffuse infiltration with histiocytes (lepromatous) (Table 1).

Table 1. Tuberculoid leprosy compared with lepromatous leprosy.

	Tuberculoid	*Lepromatous*
Immunity	High	Low
Lepromin test	Positive	Negative
Organisms	Few	Many
Infectivity	Low	High
Granulomas	Many	Absent

Tuberculoid leprosy is manifest mainly by areas of skin depigmentation, nodules on nerves, muscle paralysis and distortion resulting from nerve damage. There is a good cell-mediated reaction to the bacilli, as shown by a positive reaction to an injection of an extract of the bacilli (lepromin test). Also it is very difficult to find organisms in the lesions, which show plentiful well-developed giant cell granulomas. It is rare for patients with tuberculoid leprosy to transmit the disease to others.

At the other extreme, lepromatous leprosy shows more destructive lesions. There is a low level of immunity and the lepromin test is negative. The histiocytes contain very many bacilli but giant cell granulomas are not seen. The histiocytes (which do not acquire epithelioid characteristics) do not seem to have the capacity to kill the bacilli. Transmission of the disease occurs mainly from these cases. They do, however, develop antibodies to the bacilli, for hypergammaglobulinaemia occurs and immune complex manifestations are complications: the antibodies are ineffective, for the organisms are intracellular.

Between the two extremes is borderline leprosy and the disease can change in its pattern through this intermediate zone. An important point is that the different clinical manifestations are caused by variations in the host response rather than by differences in the infecting organisms. This is true of many disorders (e.g. tuberculosis) but it is often not as obvious as in this disease.

Syphilis is another chronic infection which shows considerable variation in its clinical manifestations. It is a venereal disease (i.e. transmitted by sexual contact) caused by a spirochaete, *Treponema pallidum*. The organisms enter through the epithelium of a mucous membrane, for example that of the glans penis. They are then quickly distributed around the body via the lymphatics and blood vessels. At this stage there is virtually no cell change or inflammation. About three weeks after infection a lesion, called a chancre, appears at the original site of entry. It is a slightly raised lesion which then ulcerates and subsequently heals. The histology of a chancre shows many lymphocytes and plasma cells. About six weeks later the lesions of secondary syphilis develop. These are very variable but painless lymphadenopathy and symmetrical mucocutaneous rashes are frequently seen, as are papules and condylomata lata (see pp. 187 and 190). These lesions are highly infectious, contain many spirochaetes and show lymphocytes and plasma cells grouped around small vessels. Ultimately these also heal and the disease enters its latent period. In about two-thirds of untreated patients no other manifestations develop, but in about one-third lesions of tertiary syphilis occur, sometimes after many years. These lesions are found in the cardiovascular and central nervous system (see Chapters 13 and 25) and also in other organs where gummas may develop. A gumma is a mass with a centre of coagulative necrosis which is surrounded by chronic inflammatory cells including histiocytes, some of which may be multinucleate; there is fibrous tissue around these cells and endarteritis is seen in adjacent vessels.

Syphilis is an intriguing disease because the organisms, though very invasive, cause little cell damage unless present in enormous numbers. The manifestations of the disease only appear after the immune system has been exposed to the organism. The lesions should therefore be considered to be, at least in part, hypersensitivity reactions. This is certainly true for those lesions seen in the tertiary stage when organisms are difficult to find but tissue damage is extensive.

The laboratory tests for diagnosis are also interesting. The organisms can be identified directly by dark ground microscopy in material taken from primary and secondary lesions. The serological tests detect antibodies in the serum. These are of two types. Historically, the first ones that could be demonstrated were not directed at the treponeme itself but at certain body constituents and were thought to develop as a result of tissue damage. These were the antibodies which were detected by such tests as the Wassermann reaction (WR) and the VDRL (Venereal Disease Reference Laboratory) test and are often called reaginic antibodies. Subsequently, tests for antibodies directed at treponemal antigens, such as the Treponema pallidum immunobilization test (TPI) or the fluorescent treponemal antibody test, have been used.

Group 2

The chronic inflammatory diseases lacking a well-marked acute phase and also lacking granulomas comprise a mixed group. Some of them are associated with abnormalities of immunity and are discussed in Chapter 4. Two examples can be mentioned here.

Cirrhosis of the liver is basically a chronic inflammatory process in an organ with a well-developed capacity for parenchymal regeneration. The commonest cause in Britain is excess alcohol consumption. This leads to parenchymal cell damage and necrosis to which the liver responds with regeneration and fibrosis. After a single insult the liver returns to normal, but in some people persistent alcohol abuse leads to the disordered nodular regeneration and fibrosis of cirrhosis which then produce portal hypertension and liver cell failure (see Chapter 17). Regeneration may becomes so disordered that a malignant tumour of the hepatocytes (a hepatoma) develops. In Britain most hepatomas develop in people with a pre-existing cirrhosis.

Chronic peptic ulcers occur in or adjacent to gastric mucosa which secretes acid and enzymes. Many factors play a part in the development, but the presence of such mucosa is a prerequisite. A breach occurs in the epithelium and an ulcer crater, with underlying inflammation, forms. The destructive elements cause this to penetrate into the wall while inflammatory and healing processes hold it in check. If destruction is rapid, then the crater can quickly enlarge and perforate through the wall into the peritoneum causing peritonitis, or into a large blood vessel causing bleeding. More usually, however, granulation tissue and fibrosis develop in the damaged muscle coat and epithelium regenerates at the edges of the ulcer. This may completely cover the crater and healing occurs, leaving a small scar, or the ulcer may persist with increasing fibrosis. If this is at the pyloric end of the stomach or in the duodenum, the contraction of the fibrous tissue brought about by the myofibroblasts can lead to narrowing of the channel and to obstruction. Microscopically, dead tissue and polymorphonuclear leucocytes are seen on the ulcer surface, with some fibrinous exudate, but immediately beneath this there is granulation tissue and then fibrosis. Chronic inflammatory cells are seen in the outer layers. Arteries close to the ulcer show intimal proliferation which may be so marked as to lead to obliteration of the lumen. This change is called endarteritis obliterans and it is very common close to sites of chronic inflammation. It can be considered helpful in that it may diminish the likelihood of a major bleed, but it can also impair the blood supply to the healing ulcer.

4

Specific Immunity and Hypersensitivity

In medicine, 'immunity' means protection from disease. Immunity to infection depends on the non-specific defences mentioned in Chapter 3and also on specific immune responses. The latter are brought about by the lymphoid system in conjunction with the mononuclear phagocytes and are initiated by antigens. Antigens are molecules that the body recognizes as 'non-self' and to which a response is mounted, mediated in part by antibodies. The modern science of immunology has grown from the study of these responses, whose major characteristics are specificity, memory and recognition of non-self. In this context, 'memory' means that the first encounter with an antigen modifies the body's subsequent responses to that antigen. This altered reactivity may lead to elimination of the antigen, when the response is described as an *immune reaction*. Sometimes the response is exaggerated or misdirected and can lead to tissue damage out of proportion to the stimulus: this is called *hypersensitivity*. These are not entirely different processes, for the mechanisms involved are the same. Normally the many checks and balances in the system produce a result favourable to the individual— that is to say, 'immunity'.

The lymphohistiocytic system

The physiology of the lymphoid system was first elucidated in experimental animals and the nomenclature used has been extrapolated to man, where the evidence supports a very similar system. There are two major groups of lymphocytes: the B lymphocytes (so called because in birds they arise from the Bursa of Fabricius) and the T lymphocytes (so called because, in animals, they can be shown to require processing by the thymus before they are able to function properly). B cells are responsible for humoral immunity: they mature to plasma cells which make and release immunoglobulins. T cells are responsible for cell-mediated immunity, which acts against intracellular organisms; they also have many controlling functions (helping and suppressing) in the immune system. By light microscopy, T and B cells look alike but they can be distinguished by markers carried on their surfaces. B

26

cells have easily demonstrated immunoglobulins on their surfaces; these are the receptors for antigens. T cells do not have easily demonstrated immunoglobulin receptors but can be recognized by the peculiar characteristic of spontaneously binding sheep red cells in vitro; the nature of the T cell receptors for antigen is still debated. The mononuclear phagocytes participate in the system both because they help to prepare some antigens for recognition by the lymphocyte system and also because they are recruited by T lymphocytes and used as effectors in cell-mediated immune reactions. Though it is of great functional complexity, the immune system can be considered to have an afferent arm, a central processing unit and an efferent arm. The afferent arm comprises those mechanisms which lead to an antigen being presented to the surface of a lymphocyte where it is recognized as 'non-self'. The processing unit comprises the changes within and between lymphocytes which lead to proliferation of cells committed to a response to the antigen. The efferent arm comprises the effector mechanisms which act against the antigen: these are mediated through humoral antibodies (B lymphocytes) and through cell-mediated reactions (T lymphocytes).

The afferent arm is concerned with presenting antigen to cells which recognize it and are then stimulated. Macrophages, especially the dendritic macrophages of the skin and lymph nodes, are particularly involved in this presentation. The spleen, lymph nodes and the mucosa associated lymphoid tissue are concentrations of cells strategically placed to screen lymph, blood and absorbed substances for their self/ non-self character. The circulating lymphocytes may also recognize antigen in other tissues and organs. Most antigen recognition and lymphocyte stimulation requires T cell involvement; only a minority of antigens directly stimulate B cells.

The *central processing* of the received information is best developed in the concentrations of lymphoid tissue. It involves transformation of the recognizing cells and proliferation of effector cells. This is seen most clearly in the lymph nodes, with expansion of the B cell areas (cortical) and the T cell areas (paracortical) of lymph nodes and the corresponding areas of the spleen. B cell responses are characterized histologically by the development of lymphoid follicles with large germinal centres; T cell responses do not have this structure.

Humoral antibodies are immunoglobulins (Fig. 1). The basic molecule is composed of four polypeptide chains linked by disulphide bonds (–S–S–). There are two central heavy chains (H) and two shorter light chains (L). Papain digestion cleaves the molecule into two Fab fragments which contain the antigen-binding sites, and an Fc portion which can activate complement and bind to receptors on monocytes. IgM is a pentamer; IgA exists partly as a dimer; IgG, IgD and IgE are monomers of the basic four-chain unit. The subclasses differ in the nature of their heavy chains but kappa or lambda light chains are found in all classes. J chains link the units of the polymer immunoglobulins.

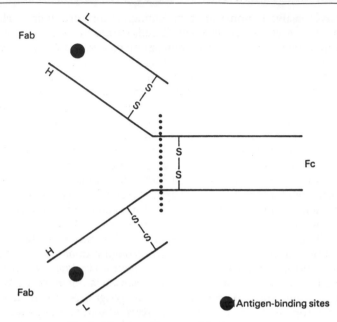

Fig. 1. Diagram of immunoglobulin monomer.

The *efferent arm* effects responses through plasma cells and T cells. Humoral antibodies produce their effects in a number of different ways, depending partly on the type of antibody, partly on the antigen, and partly on where the antigen is found. *Complement activation* frequently occurs, particularly with IgM reactions. There are at least nine major components of complement (C1–C9) and activation of the sequence classically occurs when the combination of antigen and antibody binds C1. A sort of cascade is initiated (similar in some ways to the coagulation cascade) which finishes with C9 and the lysis of cell membranes. In addition inflammatory mediators are released between C3 and C9 which have functions such as being chemotactic for polymorphs. Complement may also be activated by an alternate pathway, not involving antibody, by such substances as bacterial endotoxin. The classical and alternate pathways differ in their early steps but are the same from C3 onwards. *Opsonization* is the process by which cells are made more susceptible to phagocytosis; this is a very important function of antibody and is often brought about by immune adherence to monocytes (which have receptors for Fc on their surfaces). *Agglutination* and *precipitation* may also play a part. Toxins are *neutralized* by antibody and are then removed harmlessly from the body. IgA is secreted from mucosal surfaces and there acts as a defence; it also combines in the circulation with food antigens that have entered through the intestine—the complexes are then excreted through the liver. IgE is found on the surface of mast cells, particularly in mucous membranes. When antigen combines with IgE the mast cell degranulates, releasing its inflammatory mediators. There is evidence that this response plays a part in the defences against parasites.

Whereas immunoglobulins are particularly effective in blood and tissue fluids, the T lymphocyte effector mechanisms are very important in acting against agents that can exist within cells. T lymphocytes are necessary for the efficient production of immunoglobulin and have many regulating functions in the immune system (e.g. helper, suppressor and memory cells). There is also one subgroup of T lymphocytes which can proliferate and be directly toxic for cells bearing virus particles on their surfaces. This action is important for the containment of many diseases including mumps, measles and that caused by herpes viruses. T cells can be directly cytotoxic in other situations, but most T cell effects seem to be brought about by the production of *lymphokines*. These are polypeptide non-immunoglobulin products of lymphocytes which affect other cells, particularly monocytes. Macrophage-activating factor (MAF) enables the monocyte to kill an intracellular organism that was previously resistant to its effects; macrophage chemotactic factor brings monocytes to the area; migration-inhibition factor (MIF) keeps them there; and interferon inhibits viral replication. It is interesting that many of the actions of lymphokines are non-specific in that other organisms may be affected besides the one that initiated the response, e.g. interferon affects many viruses. The specificity of the reaction lies in the initial recognition rather than in the effector mechanism.

After the successful removal of an infectious agent, the system is primed so that exposure to that agent on a subsequent occasion leads to a secondary response which is accelerated in time and increased in quantity. The altered reactivity may be so efficient that no clinical manifestations occur on a second exposure—it is uncommon to get mumps twice. The individual can then be said to be immune to that particular disease.

The state of specific immunity can be acquired actively or passively. Active immunity occurs when the body's own cells produce the response, and can either be naturally acquired or artificially induced by immunization with an agent which has the antigenicity but not the pathogenicity of the natural organism (e.g. poliomyelitis immunization). Passive immunity is acquired by transfer of antibodies from one individual to another. This can be naturally acquired, as when antibodies are transferred across the placenta to the fetus, or artificially acquired, as in a patient receiving hyperimmune globulins from another individual (e.g. for infectious hepatitis).

Hypersensitivity is said to occur when a specific immune reaction leads to inappropriate tissue damage. An example is the skin test used to assess previous exposure to tuberculosis, originally called the Mantoux test. An extract of bacilli (purified protein derivative) is injected intradermally.

In an individual with no previous exposure there is no visible effect and no tissue damage ensues. In an individual who has had tuberculosis in the past, or who has been immunized with BCG (bacille Calmette–Guérin), a red raised area develops after 24–48 hours: this may be painful. The histology is that of a lymphocyte and monocyte infiltrate, and the reaction gradually resolves. The reaction is described as hypersensitivity because tissue damage is caused, not directly by the antigen (which is harmless in unexposed individuals), but by the immune reaction. Nevertheless, it is used in practice as a measure of immunity to tuberculosis. In occasional individuals the reaction is extreme with extensive necrosis, granuloma formation and spread to lymph nodes.

Hypersensitivity reactions were originally divided into immediate and delayed types, on the basis of their speed of onset. The early immunologists showed that the capacity for immediate-type reactions could be transferred from one individual to another by serum factors (later shown to be immunoglobulins). The capacity for delayed-type reactions could not be transferred in this way, but in animals transfer of spleen cells from a hypersensitive animal to an unexposed one could transfer the reaction. We now know that the immediate-type reactions are B cell mediated (immunoglobulin) and the delayed type are T cell dependent. Currently the most helpful classification of hypersensitivity reaction is the subdivision of the antibody-mediated group into types I, II and III, the cell-mediated group being type IV. A fifth type has also been proposed.

Type I: homocytotropic antibody mediated

Some individuals, particularly those with a family history of atopy, respond to some antigens (such as those in pollen) by the production of homocytotropic antibodies (usually IgE) which become fixed (by their Fc portions) to mast cells, rather than remaining in the circulation. The mast cells are seen particularly in mucous membranes. When antigen is then brought into contact with the antibody, the mast cell releases its mediators and sets up an inflammatory reaction. This mechanism is seen in atopic asthma, hay fever and eczema. Sometimes drug reactions or injections of foreign proteins result in anaphylaxis, which is a widely disseminated, life-threatening version of this; vascular permeability increases in many sites in the body, fluid is lost from the circulation, the blood pressure drops and death may result.

Type II: antibody-mediated cytotoxicity

In this form, antibodies (IgG or IgM) are directed at antigens on cell surfaces. When antigen and antibody unite, complement is activated and damage to the cell results. This mechanism occurs in, for example, immune haemolytic anaemias and thrombocytopenias.

Type III: immune complex disorders

Antigens and antibodies form complexes in the circulation or in the interstitial tissues. This is a common physiological occurrence and most complexes are removed from the body without damage. However, some complexes, often called toxic complexes, do cause damage. The damaging potential of complexes depends on their size, composition, ability to activate complement, and site of deposition.

The classic example of a systemic immune complex disease is serum sickness, both in the human and in the experimental animal. Following one intravenous injection of foreign protein (especially from another species), some individuals respond with an illness about two weeks later characterized by vasculitis, arthralgia, a skin rash, glomerulonephritis, and pyrexia. It has been shown that at this time the antibody titre is rising and antigen is still present in the circulation. Complexes are formed and normally removed, but if the wrong immunochemistry is present, complexes are deposited in tissues, where inflammation occurs. In the one-shot model the disease subsides as antibody level increases and antigen is eliminated, but the model can be manipulated by repeated injections to give chronic disease. Many cases of glomerulonephritis are thought to develop by similar mechanisms.

In some disorders the complexes are not in the circulation but are found locally. The experimental model of this is the local version of the Arthus phenomenon where an animal receives repeated subcutaneous injections of antigen until it develops high levels of precipitating antibody. Antigen and antibody then unite in the extracellular tissue, activate complement, release inflammatory mediators, initiate thrombosis in small vessels, and a necrotic inflammatory lesion develops. Human equivalents of this mechanism are those lung disorders in which individuals develop very high levels of precipitating antibodies to organic dusts (e.g. farmer's lung, bird fancier's lung). When the dust is inhaled the reaction is precipitated in the walls of the alveoli (extrinsic allergic alveolitis). In the acute phase there is breathlessness accompanied by an acute inflammatory reaction which may resolve completely, but repeated attacks lead to pulmonary fibrosis. A mechanism like this also occurs in the joints in rheumatoid arthritis.

Type IV: cell-mediated hypersensitivity reactions

These occur in response to many bacterial products. The example of the Mantoux test in tuberculosis has already been discussed, and similar reactions occur with other tests such as the lepromin test for leprosy.

Lymphocytes and histiocytes occur in the lesions, with giant cell granulomas developing if the antigen is not eliminated.

Type V: stimulatory hypersensitivity

This occurs when antibody combines with an antigen on a cell surface and induces stimulation of cell function. Such a situation occurs in Graves' disease, a form of hyperactivity of the thyroid gland. The stimulation may go on to damage the cells, so it is possible to view this as a variant of type II.

Collagen disease and autoimmunity

These two terms are used to indicate concepts which have been useful in the development of the understanding of immunological diseases. The term 'collagen disease' was introduced to draw attention to a group of diseases of unknown aetiology but which had in common multisystem involvement, protean manifestations and lesions occurring in connective tissue and vessels of the affected organs rather than affecting parenchymal cells. Fibrinoid necrosis was a common feature. The group included such disorders as polyarteritis nodosa, systemic lupus erythematosus (SLE), rheumatoid arthritis, systemic sclerosis and dermatomyositis. (The term was never used to include the congenital abnormalities of collagen.) Many of these disorders were subsequently shown to have associated autoimmune phenomena. The term 'autoimmunity' is used to describe the situation in which the specific immune response is directed at a self-antigen. The concept originally implied that the reaction was causing the disease, but this has had to be modified, for it is clear that in some situations tissue damage results in antibodies but that these do not cause the disease (e.g. anti-myocardial antibodies after myocardial infarction). Nowadays the term is used for those disorders in which autoantibodies are present and may be linked to the pathogenesis of the disease. What initiates these disorders is still unclear, but antibodies can play a direct part in their progress. For example, the anti-basement membrane antibody in the serum of Goodpasture's syndrome (a rare form of glomerulonephritis) fixes directly to the renal glomerular basement membrane to cause the tissue lesions. In Graves' disease the antibody to thyroid cells clearly is causing disease. Another way in which autoantibodies can be damaging is by forming immune complexes either in the circulation or in situ. The renal damage in SLE is largely produced by this mechanism. In other situations the circulating antibody may be a useful marker for diagnosis of disease but there is no good evidence that it causes the disease (for example the anti-mitochondrial antibodies in primary biliary cirrhosis). Cell-mediated immunity may also play a part in directly damaging cells. This is suspected but not proven by the appearances of the histology in pernicious anaemia where there is an atrophic gastritis with a heavy lymphoid infiltrate.

There is a spectrum of autoimmune disorders ranging from those with lesions in one organ and circulating antibodies which react with structures only found in that organ, to those affecting many organs and autoantibodies directed at many structures. Organ-specific disorders include autoimmune thyroiditis (Hashimoto's disease, Graves' disease and primary myxoedema) and pernicious anaemia with atrophic gastritis. Examples of non-organ-specific specific autoimmunity are systemic lupus erythematosus and rheumatoid arthritis. Between the two extremes are disorders in which the lesion may be localized but the antibody is non-organ specific, e.g. primary biliary cirrhosis.

Systemic lupus erythematosus is a multisystem disease occurring mainly in women. Inflammatory lesions are seen in the kidneys, joints, skin, heart and other organs. Many of the manifestations are explicable in terms of inflammation resulting from immune complex disease, for the immunological hallmark of this disease is the presence of antibodies to nuclear components. These antibodies (anti-nuclear factor, anti-DNA antibody etc.) are used in diagnosis. Several histological features can suggest the diagnosis but the only pathognomonic lesion is the haematoxyphil body, which is a deposit of altered nucleoprotein. The untreated disease has a very bad outlook but, with immunosuppression, about three-quarters of the patients survive for five years, the prognosis being largely determined by the renal and central nervous system involvement. Some strains of mice have a very similar disorder. Studies of humans and animals with similar disorders suggest that it is induced by a virus in a genetically predisposed individual, but this remains a hypothesis.

Rheumatoid arthritis is a chronic progressing inflammatory condition mainly affecting the joints but having systemic manifestations sometimes affecting subcutaneous tissue, lungs, blood vessels and other organs. In the joints the most prominent lesion initially is in the synovial membrane. It undergoes a villous proliferation and is packed with lymphocytes and plasma cells. Immune complexes are present in joint fluids; they are composed of autoantibody directed at the Fc portion of IgG. Self-associating complexes are thus produced, complement activated and inflammatory mediators released. These damage the hyaline cartilage; proliferating synovium spreads over the articular surface producing distortion and sometimes resulting in fibrous ankylosis of the joint. The serum of these patients also contains an autoantibody, 'rheumatoid factor'; this is usually an IgM anti-IgG and its detection is the basis of the serological tests for rheumatoid arthritis.

Organ transplantation

Successful transplantation of kidneys as a treatment for chronic renal failure means that this form of therapy is likely to be used more in the future. The fate of an organ graft depends partly on its antigenic relationship to the recipient. Autografts (self–self) are fully accepted, as are isografts (between genetically identical individuals of the same species). Xenografts (from another species) are strongly rejected. The usual organ graft in man is an allograft (between genetically different individuals of the same species) and its fate is variable. Because of inherited differences in the human leucocyte antigens (HLA) carried on the surface of cells of the graft, there is a tendency for the graft to be rejected. This is an action of the specific immune response and, because it is undesirable, it is regarded as hypersensitivity. The tendency to rejection may be strong or weak and the weaker responses can be overcome by immunosuppression. Hypersensitivity reactions of type II and IV are particularly frequent, but type III reactions also occur. Rapid rejection occurs when the recipient has high levels of cytotoxic antibody reacting with antigens on the endothelial cells of the graft. The more common acute rejection episode is mainly a cell-mediated reaction, when the graft becomes infiltrated with lymphoid cells. These episodes can usually be overcome by temporarily increasing immunosuppression. The long- term survival of a graft is often determined by the renal ischaemia resulting from arterial narrowing, thought to be the result of repeated minor rejection episodes.

Rejection is not the only problem for the patient with a graft. Immunosuppression brings the many problems of increased susceptibility to infection and there is also an increased incidence of neoplasia. Fortunately many grafts function very well for many years and make transplantation a rewarding therapy.

5

Pathological Reactions to Virus Infections

Viruses are obligate intracellular parasites which depend for their metabolic processes upon the host cell. They contain only one type of nucleic acid, either deoxyribonucleic acid (DNA) or ribonucleic acid (RNA), in contrast to all other living cells which possess both. This nucleic acid (the viral genome) is surrounded by a protein sheath referred to as the capsid and in some viruses there is a further covering envelope which contains lipid. The complete virus particle is known as a virion and it shows a symmetry which may be cubical, helical or complex. The classification of viruses is not universally agreed, but a suggested classification is based on the type of viral nucleic acid (DNA or RNA), the presence or absence of an envelope covering the capsid, and the type of symmetry shown by the virus.

Growth of viruses

Since they depend on host cells for their metabolic activity, viruses cannot be grown on culture media in the same way as bacteria. They need living cells for their propagation and hence are usually grown in tissue culture. The chemical code contained within the nucleic acid of the virus induces the host to synthesize identical molecules of viral nucleic acid and protein from which viral particles are assembled. Viral particles released from damaged cells are adsorbed on the specific sites on the surface of further cells. This adsorption depends on the specificity of receptors in the protein coat of the virus and it is probable that the predilection of viruses for certain types of cells depends on the specificity of the reaction sites (and these may be HLA dependent). Cells which allow the growth of viruses inside them are called permissive; those which do not allow this multiplication are called non-permissive. Following attachment to the surface of a cell, the nucleic acid is stripped off the capsid and envelope and enters the cell. There, it induces a permissive cell to synthesize viral molecules which are assembled into virions and then shed.

Cellular changes of viral infection

When viruses are grown in tissue culture their observed effect on the cultured cells is known as a cytopathic effect. In vivo the changes seen with a virus infection are due to the direct effect of the virus on the cells in which it is growing and also due to the accompanying inflammation. Viruses have no direct effect on non-permissive cells. Their effect on permissive cells varies from the production of rapid and extensive destruction to having no visible result. Rapid destruction of cells is most often seen with acute viral illnesses, such as hepatitis A where focal necroses with an accompanying inflammatory reaction are seen in the liver; other cells which contain virus may show degenerative changes such as swelling and vacuolation. Inclusion bodies are seen with some virus infections. These are intracellular accumulations of virus particles, either in the nucleus or in the cytoplasm, or both. Intracytoplasmic inclusions are seen, for example, in chronic hepatitis B (ground glass cells) vaccinia (Guarnieri bodies) or rabies (Negri bodies). Intranuclear inclusions are seen with herpes simplex, chicken pox and cytomegalovirus infection. Multinucleate cells often form as a result of cell fusion: a good example of this is the Warthin–Finkeldey giant cells which are seen in lymphoid tissue in measles. Some viruses have an extremely long incubation period, measured in years. These are known as slow viruses and were first described in animals. Some examples have been described in the central nervous system in man, e.g. in Jakob–Creutzfeld disease degeneration of neurons is present when the process is fully developed but nothing is seen during the very long incubation period. Persistent viruses are those which do have an acute phase but instead of being eliminated become dormant (like herpes simplex or zoster in ganglion cells) and only produce visible lesions when they are reactivated. Cellular proliferation is produced by some viruses. It is seen in man in, for example, the squamous papillomas produced by the common wart virus. In animals, truly malignant tumours are produced by viruses and this oncogenic effect may play a part in some human malignancies. Recent evidence shows that some genes, associated with apparently normal cells, may be related to the formation of tumours. If these *oncogenes* are incorporated into the viral genome, they are capable of transferring this tumorigenic effect to other cells. Inflammatory reactions which accompany viral infections are usually characterized by lymphocytes, plasma cells and histiocytes, rather than by polymorphonuclear leucocytes. If there is a leucocytosis in the bloodstream, it is usually lymphocytic.

Immune response to virus infections

Different parts of the virion can be antigenic and stimulate a specific immunological reaction. This may involve humoral antibodies and/or a cell-mediated response. Neutralizing and complement-fixing antibodies can often be demonstrated, but they are only useful in defence if the virus is accessible: they do not act on the intracellular phase. Humoral antibodies are therefore particularly important in preventing second infections of a virus which has an extracellular phase. Cell-mediated responses enable the individual to deal with intracellular infections. One of the effector mechanisms is the production of lymphokines; interferon is an important one as far as viruses are concerned. Interferons are antiviral substances produced by lymphocytes or monocytes and enable susceptible cells to become non-permissive for viral growth. Another effector mechanism is the production of T lymphocytes which are cytotoxic for cells bearing viral antigens on their surfaces. Interestingly, this capacity is dependent not only on recognition of the viral antigen by the T lymphocyte, but also on the recognition of the HLA type of infected cell (i.e. the response is MHC restricted—see p. 62). The importance of T cell responses in recovery from viral infections is apparent when the severity of viral illnesses in patients with impaired T cell function is remembered. Occasionally stimulation of the specific immune response by a virus produces a hypersensitivity state, e.g. subacute sclerosing panencephalitis with measles or chronic active hepatitis with hepatitis B virus.

6

Protozoal and Helminthic Infections

Protozoa and metazoa cause disease most frequently in tropical rather than in temperate countries. This is due partly to climatic factors and partly to the lower levels of public health and hygiene which exist in the Third World. In nature there are many hundreds of species of protozoa and potentially parasitic metazoa but relatively few are capable of infecting man. These few are the ones which have evolved mechanisms for overcoming the host defences.

Protozoa

Amoebiasis

This is caused by the swallowing of cysts of *Entamoeba histolytica*. The cyst wall is resistant to the acid gastric juices but dissolves in the alkaline intestinal secretion to release the vegetative form. These amoebae may occur in the lumen of the bowel where they do not necessarily give rise to infection, or they may penetrate the mucosa of the large intestine to produce local necrosis and flask-shaped ulcers. Characteristically there is little accompanying inflammation, the necrosis being mostly chemical in nature. The ulcers rarely penetrate the muscle coat of the colon. Amoebae are carried in the portal venous system to the liver where they may cause either a diffuse *amoebic hepatitis* or a local *amoebic abscess*. These abscesses may rupture into the peritoneal cavity, the right pleural cavity or the lung.

Entamoeba histolytica must be distinguished from *Entamoeba coli* which is a gut commensal. *Entamoeba histolytica* in the vegetative form ingests red cells whereas *Entamoeba coli* does not; in the encysted form, *Entamoeba histolytica* has one to four nuclei and *Entamoeba coli* up to eight nuclei. *Entamoeba coli*, being a gut commensal does not penetrate the gut mucosa and so is not found in the tissues in histological sections.

Malaria

This disease occurs most frequently in tropical and subtropical climates. There are four forms of parasite, *Plasmodium vivax* (benign tertian malaria), *P. falciparum* (malignant tertian) *P. malariae* (quartan) and *P.*

ovale (similar to benign tertian malaria). The parasites enter the circulation of man by the bite of an infected *Anopheles* mosquito and there set up the asexual cycle. The introduced *sporozoite* travels to the liver where it remains for seven days, developing into *merozoites*. These are released into the bloodstream and enter the red blood cells; here they pass through the developing stages of *trophozoite, schizont* and *merozoite*, which are released by rupture of the red cell to repeat the cycle. The release of the merozoites corresponds with the pyrexial phase—48 hours for tertian and 72 hours for quartan malaria. The sexual phase occurs by some of the merozoites developing into *micro-* (male) and *macro-* (female) *gametocytes*. When the mosquito bites an infected man, these gameto-cytes are taken with the blood into the mosquito's stomach where they mature to form *gametes*. After fertilization, they form the *zygote* which penetrates the stomach wall to form an *oocyst*. *Sporozoites* develop in the oocyst, now called a *sporocyst*, and rupture of this releases sporozoites into the body cavity of the mosquito. These sporozoites invade the mosquito salivary gland and from there are injected into man to repeat the asexual cycle.

Repeated rupture of red cells may give rise to anaemia, and the phagocytosis of parasites by the reticuloendothelial system results in enlargement of the liver, spleen and lymph nodes. Plugging of the cerebral vessels by parasite-laden red cells may give rise to congestion, small haemorrhages, and focal areas of softening of the brain—*cerebral malaria*. A sudden destruction of red cells may cause haemoglobinuria and jaundice, the latter because the liver is unable to cope with the sudden load of bilirubin resulting from the haemolysis—*blackwater fever*.

Leishmaniasis

Three forms of leishmaniasis occur.

1. *Cutaneous leishmaniasis*, or *oriental sore*, is caused by *L. tropica*, a round or oval organism, about 2 μm in diameter, found particularly in histiocytes in the lesions. It is transferred from a lesion to the new host by a sandfly and causes a skin sore which lasts for weeks or months. The disease is found particularly in the Middle East and Far East.

2. *Mucocutaneous leishmaniasis*. The lesions, which are similar to those of cutaneous leishmaniasis, affect mucous membranes as well as the skin. The causative organism is *L. braziliensis* and the disease occurs in South America.

3. *Kala-azar*, caused by *L. donovani*, is also spread by sandflies. There is proliferation of the reticuloendothelial system causing hepato-splenomegaly and lymphadenopathy. Phagocytic cells in the bone marrow, lungs, gastrointestinal system, kidneys and skin are numerous and contain many parasites. The disease occurs in Africa and Asia. The

massive splenomegaly may be associated with depression of haemo-poiesis in the bone marrow resulting in pancytopenia.

Trypanosomiasis

This disease is also known as sleeping sickness. *Trypanosoma gambiense* and *T. rhodesiense* are carried by the tsetse fly. They are slender, flagellate organisms about 15 μm in length and up to 3 μm in width. The infection causes cerebral oedema, minute haemorrhages and microinfarcts. There is also lymph node hyperplasia and often hepatosplenomegaly. A different variety of trypanosomiasis to that found in Africa occurs in Central and South America (Chagas' disease, caused by *T. cruzi*).

Toxoplasmosis

Toxoplasma gondii, a crescent-shaped protozoon about 5 μm in length, causes two types of disease, *congenital toxoplasmosis* associated with transplacental infection and *adult toxoplasmosis*. Congenital toxoplasmosis may result in hydrocephalus, cerebral calcification, choroidoretinitis, pneumonitis and myocarditis. Adult toxoplasmosis causes a disease similar to infectious mononucleosis (glandular fever) but with a negative Paul–Bunnell test. The disease can be confirmed by the characteristic lymph node appearances in which there are focal collections of histiocytes giving rise to granulomas of distinctive appearance. Rarely, it may cause pulmonary and cerebral infection in adults. A rising *dye test* titre and *fluorescent antibody* titre are diagnostic of recent infection.

Others

Trichomonas vaginalis is a flagellate protozoon which occurs in Britain and is a relatively common causes of vaginitis and urethritis. *Giardia lamblia* is a similar flagellate protozoon which inhabits the small intestine and sometimes causes the malabsorption syndrome. Both organisms live on the epithelial surface and, though inflammation is seen, it is seldom that the organisms invade tissue.

Helminths

Tapeworms (cestodes)

Man is the definitive host for three types of tapeworm: *Taenia saginata* (beef tapeworm), *T. solium* (pork tapeworm) and *Diphyllobothrium latum* (fish tapeworm), the last of which is less important in the United Kingdom than the other two worms. Cattle or pigs eat the ova of the tapeworm passed in human faeces. The ova develop into embryos in the animal intestinal tract and these embryos enter the bloodstream and become encysted in the tissues. When uncooked, or inadequately cooked meat containing ova is eaten, the ova develop into worms in the human intestine. The head, or scolex, is necessary for the survival of the worm. It is attached to the jejunum by four suckers. The eggs develop in the segments of the worm called proglottids, and these are shed in the faeces. The fish tapeworm is sometimes associated with a megaloblastic anaemia.

Cysticercosis is a disease caused by the ingestion by man of the ova of *T. solium*. These ova hatch in the upper intestine and the larvae penetrate the mucosa to enter the mesenteric vessels. After passing through the lungs, the larvae give rise to systemic infection. Each larva develops into a thin-walled cyst—cysticercus—and there is surrounding inflammation. When the worm dies, the cyst is replaced by dense fibrous tissue and calcification. These cysts can form in the brain, and their presence there is one of the causes of epilepsy.

Hydatid disease is caused by infestation by *Echinococcus granulosus* (*T. echinococcus*), the dog tapeworm. The eggs are excreted in the faeces of the dog and are ingested by man, cow, sheep or pig. The eggs hatch in the upper intestine and the embryos penetrate the bowel wall to enter the bloodstream. They may be disseminated anywhere in the body. Man may be infected directly in this way or indirectly by eating contaminated meat containing the embryos. When they lodge in the tissues (the common sites being the liver, lung, brain and bone), the embryos develop into hydatid cysts possessing an outer fibrous capsule and an inner germinal layer. From this inner layer, daughter cysts, or 'brood capsules', develop and contain scolices of the young worm. The cycle is completed by a dog eating the tissues from infected animals.

The hydatid cysts may be up to 25 cm in diameter, surrounded by an inflammatory reaction containing many eosinophils. Rupture of the cyst results in secondary cysts and possibly in an anaphylactic reaction. The diagnosis may be established by a positive *complement fixation test* or by cutaneous reaction to the intradermal injection of sterile hydatid fluid (*Casoni test*).

Nematodes

Roundworms

Ascaris lumbricoides are similar to earthworms in appearance. They cause a disease known as *ascariasis*. Eggs produced in the human intestine are passed in the faeces. They undergo a period of development in the soil before being ingested. The embryos hatch in the small intestine and pass through the bowel wall into the bloodstream. They are carried to the lungs where they set up an allergic pneumonitis. From the lungs they pass up into the major air passages and from there down into the oesophagus to the intestine to complete the cycle.

Hookworm

Ancylostoma duodenale is very much smaller than *Ascaris lumbricoides*, measuring only about 1 cm in length. However, each worm can ingest between 0.5 ml and 1 ml of blood each day so that heavy infestation may cause severe iron deficiency anaemia in the host. The ova are passed in the faeces and the embryos hatch in the soil. They gain entrance to the body through the skin and pass to the lungs. From here they pass via the air passages and the oesophagus to the small intestine. The worm attaches itself to the mucosa of the upper small intestine, resulting in mucosal oedema and surrounding eosinophilic infiltration. During passage through the lungs, the parasites may cause alveolar haemorrhages and bronchopneumonia.

Threadworm

The ova are deposited around the anus and they are transferred to a new host by faecal contamination. They can frequently be found beneath the fingernails of children. The ova mature in the intestine into adult worms, the male measuring 5 mm and the female 10 mm in length. The commonest symptom is pruritus which is caused by the migrating worms depositing ova. Adult worms are frequently seen in appendicectomy specimens, particularly in children.

Trichinella

Trichinella spiralis is a worm measuring up to 5 mm in length. Man is infected most commonly by eating infected, inadequately cooked pork containing encysted larvae. These larvae develop into adult worms in the stomach and upper small intestine. The female penetrates the intestinal mucosa and deposits ova in the submucosa. The larvae which develop from these ova enter lymphatics and, after passing through the lungs, enter the systemic circulation causing infection of skeletal and cardiac muscle. Initially the larvae cause inflammation of the muscle with many eosinophils but later the larvae become encysted and surrounded by a thick fibrous capsule.

Toxocara

This is a common intestinal worm of cats and dogs, being particularly common in puppies. Its importance in man is that the ingested ova develop in the small intestine into larvae which penetrate the mucosa and enter the bloodstream. The larvae cause granulomas in the eye and brain and may also give rise to widespread inflammation of the eye leading to blindness. The larvae do not develop into adult worms in man.

Filariasis

This infection is due to *Wuchereria bancrofti*, a thread-like worm measuring up to 10 cm in length. A *Culex* mosquito takes up the larvae or microfilaria with the blood of an infected patient. The larvae penetrate the gut wall of the mosquito and, after undergoing maturation in the thoracic muscles of the mosquito, they pass down the mosquito proboscis to be injected into the skin of man during a further mosquito bite. From the skin, the larvae pass in the lymphatics to the regional lymph nodes and mature in these sites. After mating of the male and female worms, numerous microfilariae are produced by each female. These gain entrance to the bloodstream, through the lymphatic channels, the release of microfilariae occurring at night. Death of the worms causes a granulomatous reaction which results in lymphatic obstruction and chronic lymphoedema. The affected parts become grossly enlarged and the skin thickened—*elephantiasis*.

Trematodes (flukes)

Schistosomiasis

This is the most important infestation due to flukes in man. There are three species of *Schistosoma*: *S. haematobium* (bladder), *S. mansoni* and *S. japonicum* (intestinal and visceral). The eggs are passed in urine or faeces into fresh water, and hatch into larval forms (*miracidia*) which infect fresh-water snails. After a period of development in the snail they emerge as *cerceriae*. These penetrate the human skin during bathing or swimming and enter the bloodstream. They pass through the pulmonary circulation and from there enter the portal system where they mature into adult flukes. The parasites lay their eggs in the liver, intestine and bladder where they set up a granulomatous reaction. In the liver this is mainly in the portal tracts and gives rise to a 'pipe-stem' fibrosis. In the bladder there is hyperplasia of the lining mucosa which may progress to carcinoma.

7

Circulatory Disturbances

Haemorrhage

When blood has leaked out from a blood vessel, a haemorrhage is said to have occurred. If the leak is small and is from a capillary, it is called *petechial*. *Purpura* is said to exist if a collection of petechial haemorrhages occurs in the skin or the mucous membranes. If a larger haemorrhage develops in subcutaneous tissue, this is called an *ecchymosis*, or *bruise*. When the haemorrhage is so substantial that a lump of clotted blood forms, this is termed a *haematoma*.

When there has been a haemorrhage in an organ or tissue, the extravasated blood clots and is eventually broken up, the components usually being removed to other sites in the body. The red colour of the shed blood (haemoglobin) becomes transformed to a mixture of yellow and brown (chiefly bilirubin and haemosiderin) before fading, thus bringing about the characteristic features of a bruise. When a haemorrhage is very large, or when it occurs in relatively avascular areas like fibrous tissue, it may not be cleared up completely, in which case the affected area will remain brown to the naked eye and will show under the microscope the presence of many haemosiderin-containing macrophages (siderocytes) in the fibrous tissue with foreign body giant cells, often in relation to diamond-shaped clear spaces. The latter are due to cholesterol crystals from the extravasated serum which are dissolved out of the tissue in the preparation of the section.

Haemorrhages develop (a) because there is a defect in the vessel wall, or (b) because the ability of the blood to seal off breaches in the wall has become less effective than normal.

Defects of vessel wall

1. The most obvious way in which a vessel wall may become disrupted is by *trauma*. When a vessel has been cut completely through, the cut ends quickly retract; because of the greater amount of elastic tissue and smooth muscle, an artery will contract more strongly than a vein. However, the contraction closing the breach in the arterial wall will be opposed by the blood pressure tending to keep it open, with the result that blood will continue to spurt out unless assistance is given to close the

hole. This aid will, in an emergency, be by direct pressure on the cut end, or by use of a torniquet if a limb vessel is involved, or by suturing the cut end as during an operation. The blood pressure in the veins is much lower than in the arteries so that blood loss from a cut vein can be more easily controlled.

2. The vessel wall may rupture because it contains a *structural weakness*, and this is more likely in an artery than in a vein. The weakness may be due to a congenital deficiency of the wall (see p. 115), or may arise as a result of disease, such as syphilis (see p. 23). The result in both cases is fibrous replacement of the normal muscle and elastic tissue of the wall. In an artery the fibrous tissue stretches as it is inelastic and because of the pulsatile expansion, so that the vessel becomes dilated at this point; this dilatation is called an aneurysm. When the dilatation affects the whole circumference of an artery, it is termed a *fusiform* aneurysm. If only a part of the circumference is involved, then the aneurysm is *saccular*. When an aneurysm is the result of direct infection of the vessel wall, it is termed a *mycotic* aneurysm. The fibrous wall of the aneurysm is liable, in the course of time, to become so thin that blood will start to leak through the wall, or the vessel will rupture with a sudden outpouring of blood. These are examples of true aneurysms. A *false aneurysm* results from traumatic rupture of the arterial wall with the formation of a periarterial haematoma. This becomes walled off by organizing fibrous tissue but remains in communication with the arterial lumen.

3. A third way in which a vessel wall may leak blood is through *increased permeability of the endothelial lining*. The leak in these circumstances is more likely to be from capillaries (petechiae) than from thick-walled vessels. The immediate cause of increased permeability of the lining cells is not always clear. Anoxia from any cause is a frequent reason, and bacterial toxins or chemical poisons may bring it about. Dietary lack of vitamin C is a well-known reason which leads to the condition of *scurvy*, but this is no longer common in Britain because of the relatively high standard of nutrition which exists.

Defects in the blood

Spontaneous haemorrhages are liable to occur if the number of blood platelets falls to a low level (*thrombocytopenia*) or if an abnormality develops in the coagulation mechanism, as for example in haemophilia. Thrombocytopenia leads to purpura, which shows that the integrity of the capillary endothelium must be partly dependent on the number of circulating platelets. The platelets exert their haemostatic effect in two ways. They clump together and seal off breaches that may develop in the capillary wall, and they have a vasoconstrictive action as a result of the 5-hydroxytryptamine (serotonin) which is present on their surface.

Defects in the blood coagulation mechanism do not usually lead to purpura but to a diffuse and persistent oozing of blood. This may develop spontaneously or become evident as a result of a traumatic episode such as dental extraction which would be quickly followed by normal haemostasis in a normal person.

Another cause of bleeding is abnormal fibrinolysis. Normally there exists a system whereby small amounts of fibrin are destroyed by the proteolytic enzyme *plasmin*. In certain disease states the fibrinolytic system becomes abnormally activated so that it not only destroys fibrin as it forms, but it also destroys fibrinogen, resulting in a coagulation defect.

Thrombosis

The endothelial lining of the blood vessels consists normally of a smooth surface which enables the blood within to circulate without appreciable coagulation taking place. Once the endothelial lining becomes roughened, as for example following trauma, a chain of events takes place in the blood which leads to the formation of a solid mass of tissue at the roughened area, the primary purpose of which is to repair the breach in the endothelium. This mass, which is formed from the elements in the blood, is termed a *thrombus*. The first thing to happen at the damaged endothelial surface is the formation of a mass of clumped platelets. These elements will always adhere to roughened surfaces and, when adherent, will alter in texture so that they become more sticky and more amorphous. This platelet clump is of pale colour to the naked eye and is commonly termed a *white thrombus*. This appears to be all that is necessary to seal off small wounds of vascular endothelium, the platelets' surface being quickly covered by endothelial cells proliferating from the surrounding intact endothelium. The endothelial spread is very rapid in normal circumstances. If the damaged area is extensive, the white thrombus will continue to grow into the lumen of the vessel in a spiral fashion. This will create eddies in the flowing blood, which enables the concentration of blood thromboplastin to build up to a sufficiently high level to initiate the precipitation of fibrin on to the surface of the platelets. The fibrin network enmeshes red cells among the fibres and provides a roughened surface for more platelet deposition, with the result that the thrombus may become so big as to occlude the lumen of the vessel. This *red thrombus*, when seen macroscopically, will appear a dull chocolate brown with paler brown ribbing—the lines of Zahn—and can be fairly easily broken up. Under the microscope, the characteristic picture is one of alternate layers of hyaline pale-pink platelet thrombus and of darker pink fibrin fibrils surrounding red cells. The white cells chiefly palisade the platelet layers, but may also be scattered through the fibrin network.

Factors influencing thrombus formation

Important factors which favour the production of red thrombi are damaged endothelium, slowing of the circulation, and increased coagulability of the blood (Virchow's triad).

Damaged endothelium

The significance of this has already been discussed. The changes in the endothelium may be traumatic, as in crush injuries or from suture material in vascular surgery, or the damage may result from the injection of irritating chemicals. Anoxia is also an important factor in veins. In arteries, atheroma and mechanical stresses are the commonest causes of endothelial damage.

Slowing of the circulation

Whenever platelet thrombi start to form, the normal coagulation process is always initiated, but if the flow of blood is fast, the blood thromboplastin which is formed is swept away and diluted in the process. In addition, these small amounts will be neutralized by the natural anticoagulant substances which circulate in the blood. It is for this reason that red thrombi only develop slowly in arteries. In veins, by contrast, the flow is normally slow and becomes even slower under certain clinical conditions, such as congestive cardiac failure, or locally in varicose veins. The flow of blood in the deep veins of the leg is largely dependent on the pumping action of the leg muscles during exercise. The inactivity associated with lying in bed will thus slow the venous flow in the legs, and this occurs particularly if the patient is so ill that he does not move around much. Thus it is not surprising that red thrombi are much commoner and more extensive in veins than arteries and that the deep leg veins are chiefly affected, especially in ill patients in bed. The slowing of the blood flow initiates a vicious circle of tendency to thrombus formation, because it damages the endothelial lining cells by making them more anoxic.

Increased viscosity of blood will also tend to reduce blood flow. This can arise either when red cells are increased relative to the plasma (polycythaemia) or when the plasma volume decreases relative to red cells (dehydration).

Increased coagulability of the blood

There is evidence that blood coagulation proceeds more quickly after operations. There is an immediate increase in numbers of platelets which may be two- or threefold. These platelets become more sticky than normal, and an increase in activity of other clotting factors has been demonstrated. Blood also tends to coagulate more easily than normal in some blood diseases, particularly in polycythaemia where platelets are often increased in numbers. The increased viscosity of the blood is a contributory factor in this disease.

Sequels of thrombosis

Resolution

Not all thrombi persist for any length of time. Platelet clumps forming a white thrombus may be broken up by phosphatases released from the vessel wall. When fibrin strands form, they may be digested by the fibrinolytic activity of either the plasma or leucocytes. Contraction of the thrombus will lead to it shrinking back to occupy only part of the lumen of the vessel.

Organization

If the thrombus is not dissolved, then organization will occur and continuity of the vascular lumen may be restored by this means. Capillaries, fibroblasts and histiocytes move in from the intima of the vessel in order to digest and remove the components of the blood which form the thrombus and to replace it with varying amounts of fibrous stroma. The endothelial cells spread over and cover the organizing thrombus on its luminal side. Thus the thrombus which only partially occludes the lumen ends up as a fibrous plaque in the wall of the vessel covered by endothelium. The thrombus which occludes the lumen completely becomes penetrated by capillaries growing in from the vessel wall. These gradually dilate so that they establish continuity at a number of points, and the organized occlusive thrombus tends more often than not to have a number of small channels rather than a single one. It follows that this reconstructed blood vessel will be less efficient than normal.

Effects on the part supplied by the blood vessel

The effect of thrombus formation on the part supplied by a vessel will depend on whether this is the only vessel of supply to the part or whether it anastomoses with other channels which can take over its function if it is blocked. Individual arteries may, in certain situations, be the only vessels of supply—the so-called *end-arteries*—but veins are virtually never end-veins. Examples of end-arteries are seen in the brain, heart, spleen, kidney and retina.

Another factor which will determine the effect on the part is the speed of the narrowing of the lumen by the thrombus. If a thrombus forms rapidly in an end-artery, the blood supply is suddenly cut off from the part supplied and its component cells will die. Necrosis of tissue ensuing under such conditions is referred to as an *infarct*. If a thrombus forms more slowly in an artery or only partly occludes the vessel lumen, then the reduction of blood supply to the tissue supplied will take place slowly and may never be complete. This will lead to death or atrophy of a few cells at a time, and to *replacement fibrosis*. The fibrosis is often more limited than might be expected because the neighbouring unaffected vessels have had time to form anastomotic channels and thus to take over some of the blood supply to the part.

When a vein is rapidly occluded by a thrombus, the effect on the part supplied will depend on the adequacy of the collateral circulation which is, in most instances, good. In these circumstances the most that will take place will be a transient congestion and oedema of the part. On those occasions when the collateral circulation is inadequate, the affected tissue becomes engorged with blood and the circulation will cease, leading to infarction of the tissue (venous infarction). Such an event is more likely to occur with a pedunculated organ such as the testis, where torsion may cause venous obstruction leading to thrombosis and infarction.

Thromboembolism

Thrombi are friable unless they are undergoing organization, so that fragments are liable to break off into the bloodstream and embolize. Arterial emboli are rarely large, but if they lodge in those organs supplied by end-arteries, such as the spleen, kidney, heart and brain, they will lead to the formation of infarcts. Venous emboli can be very large. When a small vein, such as one of the intramuscular branches in the leg, becomes occluded by thrombus, the blood becomes stationary in the vessel on either side of the block and so will coagulate. That in the distal portion will eventually organize, but the clot attached to the thrombus in the proximal part of the vein often extends to the junction with another vessel in which there is continuing flow. At this point, further thrombus may form until the next vessel is occluded and coagulation then extends to a further tributary. In this way a long 'propagated thrombus' forms, attached to the vessel wall only in short segments. The free end of the 'propagated thrombus' will be buffeted by the blood flowing freely from the patent tributaries and is liable to be broken off, to be transported through the right side of the heart into the pulmonary artery system. Here it may block the major branches of the pulmonary artery and cause sudden death, or it may block more peripheral branches. The effects will then depend on the adequacy of the collateral circulation in this area. If this is impaired, pulmonary infarction will ensue.

Embolism

An embolus is a particulate mass which is transported in the blood and which becomes impacted in a blood vessel. It was seen in the previous section that a detached fragment of thrombus from a vessel wall is a cause of embolism in blood vessels. Emboli from thrombosed veins, reaching the pulmonary artery tree, assume great importance in clinical medicine because of the fatal outcome associated with the larger ones. The veins most frequently involved are the deep veins of the legs, the next most frequently affected are those draining the pelvic organs. The deep veins of the legs are liable to thrombose when the muscles are inactive, and this situation is most likely to arise when a patient lies in bed for any length of time. The pelvic veins become thrombosed after operations on pelvic organs, when trauma and infection may be important initiating factors. Common arterial emboli are detached fragments of atheromatous plaques. Those which break away from plaques in the carotid arteries are now considered to be a common cause of recurrent cerebral infarction.

Emboli arise from other sources as well as from thrombi in vessel walls; examples follow.

1. Vegetations on the heart valves or adjacent endothelial surfaces. Those most likely to fragment are the vegetations of either subacute or acute bacterial endocarditis. The former differ from the latter in that the infarcts which follow embolization are not liable to become septic.

2. Thrombi on the endocardial surfaces of the ventricles, particularly the left ventricle. The most common cause of these is an underlying myocardial infarct.

3. Thrombi in the atrial appendages. These are liable to develop in the fibrillating heart, as in chronic rheumatic heart disease and thyrotoxicosis.

4. Neoplastic emboli. Fragments of malignant tumour are liable to infiltrate venous channels and then break off to lodge elsewhere in the body. This mechanism is of great importance in the spread of malignant tumours.

5. Fat emboli. These are most likely to occur after a fracture of bone. Fat from the fatty marrow finds its way into the ruptured venous sinuses and gets transported to the pulmonary capillaries and through them to other tissues in the body such as the brain.

6. Air emboli. Air may be transported along veins to the heart. This can happen after superficial wounds to the veins of the neck, when the negative pressure produced by breathing sucks the air in. It is also a complication of faulty transfusion technique. A large quantity of air has to be sucked in before ill-effects are observed, and these arise as a result of frothing of blood in the right ventricle leading to obstruction of blood flow into the lungs. Caisson disease is closely related to air embolism. Inert gases, such as nitrogen, dissolve in the blood under the high pressure of air breathed by divers. If the pressure is rapidly reduced, this nitrogen bubbles out of solution giving gas emboli and the clinical effects of 'the bends'.

7. Amniotic embolism may occur during labour and gives rise to respiratory distress or coagulation abnormalities, including defibrination due to the thromboplastic activity of the amniotic fluid.

8. Parasite emboli may block small vessels such as the cerebral vessels in malaria (p. 38).

Results of embolism

Some of the effects have already been mentioned in the section on thrombosis. Emboli arising from the left atrium or ventricle, or from the mitral and aortic valves, or from the arterial lumina, will be propagated further into the arterial tree until they impact. Whether clinical effects will arise from such impaction will depend on the size of the particle and the state of the collateral circulation. If effects do become evident, these are most likely to be due to infarction of the organ involved. Sites where symptoms are liable to become manifest are the brain (e.g. hemiplegia), the kidney (haematuria) and the spleen (splenic pain). A large detached thrombus becoming wedged across the bifurcation of the aorta is called a 'saddle' embolus. This is usually of intracardiac origin and requires urgent surgical removal if the legs are to be saved.

Emboli arising in the veins are propagated to the lungs and liver. As thrombi are most likely in leg or pelvic veins, the lungs are the organs most liable to receive thrombotic emboli. The effects in the lungs will depend on the size of the emboli, and the circulatory state of the lungs. The largest emboli will impact in the main pulmonary arteries and will cause death within a few seconds as a result of the sudden cut-off of blood supply to the lungs and beyond. The smallest emboli may produce no symptoms. Intermediate ones will usually produce pulmonary infarcts, and the size of these will depend on whether or not there is pulmonary venous congestion. The more congested the lung, the larger will the infarct be following occlusion in any one situation in the pulmonary artery tree. When lungs are not congested, the blood supply through the bronchial artery system may be sufficient to maintain the proper nutrition of the lung involved by the embolus.

If thrombotic emboli are infected, abscesses are liable to develop at the site of impaction (pyaemic abscesses). This occurs in septic thrombophlebitis, in portal pyaemia, and in acute bacterial endocarditis. When malignant cells embolize, they may either die or continue to grow where impacted, and form masses of secondary growth or metastases. The conditions which favour the continued growth of neoplastic emboli are little understood. Only a small proportion of disseminated malignant cells become metastases, and the latter are more common in certain organs than others.

Ischaemia

The tissues of the body are completely dependent on an adequate supply of oxygenated blood for their proper nutrition. Whenever this supply becomes inadequate, the tissue is said to become *ischaemic*. The more active tissues suffer earlier from lack of oxygen (anoxia) than the less active. For example, epithelial cells are more susceptible than the connective tissues, and the neurons of the brain are the most susceptible of all cells, some of which will show evidence of functional disturbances after only a few seconds of oxygen deprivation. It is clear, therefore, that the effect of ischaemia on the tissues of the body will depend on, (a) the extent of tissue exposed to anoxia, (b) the susceptibility of the part to anoxia, (c) the severity of the anoxia, and (d) the duration of the anoxia.

The anoxia may be general or local. *General anoxia* is brought about when there is inadequate gaseous exchange in the lungs (such as in cardiovascular and respiratory disease), if cellular respiration is interfered with (such as in cyanide poisoning), or if red cells can no longer effectively transport oxygen (such as in anaemia and carbon monoxide poisoning). The results of *local anoxia*, if sustained for sufficiently long, are (a) replacement fibrosis, and (b) infarction.

Replacement fibrosis

Replacement fibrosis comes about in organs submitted to persistent mild anoxia. As has already been stated, an important site for this change is in the heart. If the blood supply to the heart becomes reduced slowly as a result of atheromatous disease in the coronary arteries, the myocardial fibres will die in the affected area and be replaced by fibrous tissue which can still survive under the anoxic conditions. Similar changes can occur in the kidney (ischaemic atrophy), and in the brain (replacement gliosis).

Infarction

An infarct is a sharply defined, often wedge-shaped, area of necrosis resulting from acute and complete anoxia following obstruction to the local circulation. It has already been pointed out that this obstruction occurs when either an atheromatous artery becomes completely thrombosed, or an artery becomes impacted with an embolus, and these are the common causes of infarction. However, the obstruction can be brought about in other ways: for example, torsion or twisting of a pedicle containing the blood supply may occur in a loop of intestine (volvulus), in an ovarian cyst, or in a testicle. The infarction in these circumstances is usually haemorrhagic, because the veins become more easily obstructed than the arteries. Accidental infarction may be brought about by ligature of an artery at operation.

When a vessel lumen is obstructed, the extent of infarction of the tissue involved will depend on the blood supply to the area. If sufficient collateral blood channels exist, the tissue is much less likely to become necrotic than otherwise. The liver and lungs are two organs which receive a double blood supply so that if these organs are otherwise normal, occlusion of a branch of one of the vessels may produce no change. However, infarcts become a common complication in the lung if the circulatory system is abnormal, as in congestive cardiac failure. In the heart, kidney, spleen and brain, collateral circulations are not normally so well developed, so that infarcts more easily develop. In the case of the heart, the slowly progressive narrowing which occurs in the atheromatous arteries tends to open up channels of communication between neighbouring branches, so that infarcts are often smaller than expected following the occlusion of an atheromatous artery.

The changes of infarction are exemplified by those occurring in myocardial infarction (p. 100) and in the kidney. If an interlobular artery of the kidney is occluded, a wedge-shaped infarct develops with its base on the capsular surface and the apex at the occluded vessel. Initially the infarcted zone is congested because of retrograde venous filling of the anoxic capillaries. Fluid escapes from the vessels to produce oedema. Anoxia of the tissues, which undergo coagulative necrosis, causes cloudy swelling (see p. 5) of the constituent cells. The infarct now bulges on all its external surfaces and there is compression of the anoxic capillaries which results in the infarct becoming pale. The peripheral zone is less compressed and the anoxic capillaries here remain dilated, with some escape of red blood cells to produce a haemorrhagic and congested boundary. There is gradual organization of the infarcted zone with replacement fibrosis. This fibrous tissue contracts over the succeeding weeks and months to leave a depressed fibrous scar.

In those sites where the tissue is of loose texture, as in the lung and intestine, the leakage of blood into the tissues causes them to become dark and stuffed with blood. There is no compression of damaged vessels as in solid organs, so the pallor is not seen until the infarct has organized and been replaced by scar tissue.

If the infarcted area extends to a serous surface, it will produce inflammation of this lining with fibrinous exudation. Pleurisy is a complication of pulmonary infarction, pericarditis of myocardial infarction, peritonitis of intestinal infarction, and perisplenitis of splenic infarction. In each case, except in the intestine, the inflammation will be followed by the formation of scar tissue and adhesions between the visceral and the overlying parietal membranes. The complication of peritonitis will be mentioned later.

Special consideration of infarcts at individual sites

The heart

The softening of the infarcted area may lead to rupture of the wall with the immediate formation of a haemopericardium and death from cardiac tamponade, i.e. the rise in pressure within the pericardium prevents diastolic filling of the heart and results in rapid failure. If a large infarct has healed by scar formation, a cardiac aneurysm may form in the course of time, leading again to the possibility of rupture of the wall.

A common complication of myocardial infarction is inflammation of the endocardium with the formation of a mural thrombus. Emboli from such a site form the basis of some clinical complications.

The lungs

Because of the loose texture of the lung and because infarcts of the lung are common when the organs are congested, they are usually haemorrhagic in this situation. It is often difficult at post-mortem to determine where an old infarct existed, although it may have been clinically obvious in life. This indicates that pulmonary infarcts may heal and give rise to minimal scar formation.

The brain

The softening that occurs in infarcts proceeds to liquefaction in the brain so that the end-result after the absorption of the fluid is one of cyst formation or a cuplike depression of the surface of the brain.

The intestine

The peritonitis which complicates infarction of the intestine will not normally heal, because the devitalized bowel quickly becomes infected from the faeces, and generalized peritonitis will ensue unless treatment is given. The infarcted bowel will also lead to the complication of intestinal obstruction.

The extremities

The infarcts of the extremities arise (a) in old people with severe atherosclerosis of arteries, particularly in diabetics, (b) in people showing Raynaud's phenomenon due to prolonged arterial spasm, and (c) in those whose arteries are impacted by large thrombotic emboli. With the exception of Raynaud's phenomenon, the legs are most commonly involved. The ischaemic portion of the limb becomes necrotic and commonly the skin becomes dry, shrunken and blackened (dry gangrene). There is usually a sharp line of demarcation between the dead and viable areas, often with evidence of inflammation at the line of junction. If the infarcted section becomes infected, it putrefies and the lesion is termed moist gangrene.

Congestion

A part is said to be congested when its veins and capillaries are distended with blood (hyperaemia). The congestion can be local or widespread, acute or chronic, active or passive. Active congestion results from arteriolar dilatation with an increased flow of blood through capillaries and veins. Passive congestion occurs when there is venous stasis resulting in diminished vascular flow.

Acute congestion

The common cause of acute generalized passive congestion is sudden heart failure; at post-mortem the organs will show a dark purplish discoloration, and blood will exude easily from their cut surfaces. The lungs and the liver are organs in which this change is most easily seen. The common cause of acute active, local congestion is acute inflammation ('rubor'), where (as we have seen earlier) the capillaries dilate and are filled with fast-moving blood.

Chronic congestion

Local venous congestion occurs if the draining vein is partially occluded. Total occlusion of venous drainage produces venous infarction, whereas minimal occlusion may not lead even to congestion in the affected part if collateral venous drainage is adequate. More generalized venous congestion may be systemic or portal. The cause of *systemic chronic venous congestion* is chronic heart failure, which is most likely to be due to essential hypertension (hypertensive cardiac failure), diffuse pulmonary disease (e.g. emphysema) or to chronic rheumatic heart disease (e.g. mitral stenosis). If the heart failure involves the left side of the heart, the lungs, in addition to the tissues of the rest of the body, show the features of chronic congestion.

Chronically congested *lungs*, when seen at post-mortem, are dark red, often with a brown tinge. Blood flows easily from the cut surface, and the texture appears tougher than normal. Microscopically, the capillaries are seen to be tortuous and engorged with blood, some of which will have escaped into the supporting tissues and alveolar lumens. A proportion of the red blood corpuscles will have broken down so that histiocytes containing haemosiderin will be seen in both situations. The characteristic accumulations of these cells in the alveolar lumens are commonly referred to as 'heart failure cells'. The long-standing oedema of the alveolar walls results in fibrosis. The combination of this fibrosis with haemosiderin staining results in *brown induration* of the lungs. The reduced blood flow through the lungs impairs gaseous exchange and so leads to the important symptom of shortness of breath (or dyspnoea), which is a striking feature of congestive cardiac failure.

When *portal congestion* follows heart failure or, less frequently, vein thrombosis, the liver is the seat of chronic venous congestion and shows a characteristic microscopic picture which is often termed 'nut-meg'. The cut surface consists of a regular mosaic of light and dark-brown colour. The dark areas in the centres of the lobules are due to the distended and congested centrilobular veins and adjacent sinusoids. In these areas the cords of hepatic parenchymal cells are atrophic and there may be necrotic cells. The pale areas are the surrounding normal parenchyma. In fact these may be paler than normal, either because of fatty change or due to regeneration of cells which dilutes their dark lipofuscin content by cell division. In more severe cases, the congested areas may extend to come into contact with congested areas of adjacent lobules, surrounding the pale periportal areas. This appearance is known as paradoxical lobulation. Nowadays treatment usually relieves the congestion before irreversible changes occur, but very occasionally the damage is followed by fibrosis and disordered regeneration nodules giving 'cardiac cirrhosis'.

The *spleen* responds in two different ways to chronic venous congestion according to whether it is a result of congestive cardiac failure, on the one hand, or to cirrhosis of the liver (relatively common) or thrombosis of the splenic vein (relatively rare) on the other. The differences of response are probably due to the fact that the pressure in the portal venous system is much higher and more prolonged in the latter circumstances (portal hypertension) than in the former. In congestive cardiac failure, the spleen does not increase much in size, but is much firmer and darker than normal, being somewhat inappropriately called a 'cricket-ball' spleen. It cuts very crisply and the cut surface, though very dark, retains its normal markings. Microscopically, the bright red of the red pulp contrasts strikingly with the blue islands of lymphoid tissue in malpighian corpuscles (or white pulp). With portal hypertension, the spleen enlarges, sometimes to four or five times the normal size, and the capsule may show areas of fibrinous exudate or fibrous thickening. The organ appears somewhat tough on cutting and the cut surface does not show such a marked dark discoloration as in congestive cardiac failure. The splenic pattern is even more marked, however, as a result of thickening of the fibrous trabeculae, and the cut surface may be dotted about with dark areas up to a few millimetres in diameter, which are small haemorrhages resulting from the persistent congestion (Gandy –Gamna bodies). Microscopically, the spleen of portal hypertension shows a characteristic sponge-like pattern, the widely dilated vascular channels of the red pulp having thicker walls than normal. Evidence of recurrent small haemorrhages is present, with foci of siderocytes in the red pulp and impregnation of the fibrous framework with stainable iron as well as foci of more recently shed blood.

Chronic venous congestion of the other organs does not produce striking pathological changes other than a deep purple discoloration due to engorgement of the capillaries and veins. It is, however, not hard to see that this pathological change is the basis of the disorderly function which may arise in these organs as a result of the congestion from reduced blood flow. For example, patients may have symptoms of indigestion or signs of intestinal dysfunction, and the reduced blood flow through the kidneys may lead to oliguria, proteinuria, and cast formation as well as contributing to the formation of the oedema which so often dominates the clinical manifestations of congestive cardiac failure.

Shock

Shock is a word used to describe a group of clinical conditions in which there is a widespread marked reduction of tissue perfusion. If this is prolonged, there is a generalized impairment of cellular function. Clinically the patient is pale, ashen and sweating and usually has a rapid pulse and lowered blood pressure.

There are many causes for such a state, but perhaps the commonest is hypovolaemia. This results from loss of circulating fluid either as haemorrhage or as fluid redistribution to the exterior or to some site within the body. Cardiac causes, such as myocardial infarction, are frequent. Obstruction to blood flow caused, for example, by a pulmonary embolus or haemorrhage into the pericardial sac (cardiac tamponade) produces a similar picture. Occasionally shock is neurogenic and then the pulse may be slow. Shock can also be seen in overwhelming infection (especially with Gram-negative septicaemia in which there is circulating endotoxin) or in hypersensitivity states such as anaphylaxis where there is a widespread increase in vascular permeability.

Elucidating the cause and correcting it are often difficult but, if it persists, lesions develop in several organs. Patchy necrosis of myocardial fibres occurs in the heart. Stress ulcers develop in the stomach and duodenum. Foci of necrosis, often with haemorrhage, develop in the pancreas and adrenals. The lungs become congested, oedematous and haemorrhagic and the brain becomes swollen. It is therefore not surprising that many patients suffering shock die.

8

Genetic Disorders

Chromosomes

During cell division, nuclear chromatin gathers together to form threads called *chromosomes*, each of which splits lengthwise to form two *chromatids*, joined at one point called the *centromere*. Chromosomes are composed of basic proteins (histones) and deoxyribonucleic acid (DNA). Information about the appearance of chromosomes has accumulated recently due to improved methods of tissue culture and specific staining techniques. The addition of colchicine to the culture causes arrest of cell division in metaphase so that dividing cells accumulate and their chromosomes can be studied in stained preparations. Under these circumstances the two arms of the chromatids separate, being held only by the centromere, to form the shape of the letter X. The size of the chromosomes and the position of the centromere, whether it is central or towards one pole, are constant for any particular chromosome. In the human there are 46 chromosomes made up of 22 pairs of *autosomes* and 2 sex chromosomes. In the male these sex chromosomes are referred to as X and Y, whereas in the female there are two X chromosomes. The autosomes are identifiable and the pairs numbered 1–22. Ova and spermatozoa are different from somatic cells in that they have only half the number of chromosomes, i.e. 23. The nuclei of somatic cells are called *diploid* and those of the sex cells *haploid*. If nuclei have many more than the usual number of chromosomes, such as happens with many malignant cells, they are called *polyploid*.

In normal females, a condensation of chromatin, called the *Barr body*, can be found adjacent to the inner aspect of the nuclear membrane. The number of Barr bodies is one fewer than the number of X chromosomes. This is because only one X chromosome is active, the other one being normally suppressed. This suggestion was originally made by Lyon and is known as the 'Lyon hypothesis', but it has been amply confirmed. Similar sex chromatin can be seen in polymorph leucocytes as a 'drum-stick' appendage to the nucleus. Nuclei containing sex chromatin are referred to as *chromatin positive* and those without as *chromatin negative*.

Cell division

There are two forms of cell division, *mitosis* and *meiosis*. The two chromatids held together at the centromere in the early stage of mitotic division eventually separate at the centromere and move to opposite poles of the cell where they form daughter nuclei. This process is followed by constriction of the cytoplasm so that two daughter cells form with the same number of chromosomes as the parent cell. The germ cell precursors undergo meiotic (or reduction) division which consists of two stages. In the first stage, pairs of chromosomes come to lie alongside one another. At points along each chromosome they seem to be attached to the corresponding site on the partner. It is apparently at these points that cross-over of the chromosomes occurs with exchange of chromatin material from one chromosome to another. Each chromosome then separates from its partner and they gather together to form two daughter nuclei which immediately pass into the second stage of division which is comparable with mitotic division. The full meiotic division results in four haploid nuclei. All the male cells survive as spermatozoa, but only one of the four female cells survives as an ovum. When conception takes place the spermatozoon unites with the ovum, so the newly produced cell (or *zygote*) will have 46 chromosomes, one of each of the 23 pairs coming from the father, and the other from the mother.

Abnormalities

Genetic disorders are those in which the major component in the aetiology of a disease is the individual's genetic endowment. *Hereditary disorders* are those in which the genetic abnormality is present in the parent and is transmitted to the child, but some genetic disorders, particularly chromosomal anomalies, arise during cell division and new gene change can arise by mutation. There are three patterns of genetic disorder: simple gene inheritance (Mendelian), polygenic inheritance, and chromosomal abnormalities.

Simple gene inheritance (Mendelian)

A gene occupies a specific place on a chromosome—the gene locus. As chromosomes consist of identical pairs, it follows that the genes also exist as pairs. The genes may exist in identical forms or they may differ, in which case they are known as *alleles*. An abnormal gene which produces clinical disease when only one is present is said to be *dominant*; when both members of the pair have to be abnormal for clinical disease to occur, the gene is *recessive*. When the same gene is present in both sites, an individual is said to be *homozygous* with respect to this gene; when a different gene is present at both sites, an individual is said to be *heterozygous*. Dominance and recessiveness are not absolute, for heterozygous recessives may show some detectable abnormalities and also, when a dominant gene is present in the homozygous state, the disease is more severe. Patterns of inheritance depend on whether a gene is dominant or recessive and whether it is present on the autosomes or sex chromosomes.

Autosomal dominant inheritance

The disease is clinically apparent in the heterozygous state and half the children of an affected individual will be affected, male and female equally. These are rare disorders, often involving a structural protein abnormality. Three examples are *neurofibromatosis*, *polyposis coli* and *adult polycystic kidneys*.

Autosomal recessive inheritance

The disease is only clinically apparent in the homozygous state and this usually means that both parents are carriers. There is a one in four chance of a child from such parents having the disease. Abnormal autosomal recessive genes are relatively common but the chance of them producing disease depends on the degree of inbreeding in a particular community. In Caucasians, *cystic fibrosis* is present in about 1 in 2000. In blacks, sickle cell anaemia is relatively common. The enzyme deficiency states also tend to be autosomal recessive, e.g. phenylketonuria and Tay–Sachs disease.

Sex-linked inheritance

Diseases of this type are mainly due to genes carried on the X chromosome. They may act as dominant or recessive traits in the female but in the male, with only one X chromosome, they are clinically manifest if present. Haemophilia A is an X-linked recessive and is characterized by the fact that females are carriers but it is the males who suffer the effects of clinical disease.

Polygenic inheritance

Some features of an individual, such as height, are determined not by one gene locus but by several working in concert. These characteristics tend to be continuously variable within a community and no simple Mendelian ratios are seen. Some common adult disorders probably have polygenic inheritance as an important factor in their aetiology, but the presence of diseases is also influenced by environmental factors. Hypertension, diabetes mellitus and coronary heart disease all show a familial tendency, with frequencies that suggest polygenic inheritance as part of their aetiology. Cleft palate and some forms of cardiac malformation are inherited in this way. Though the inheritance is polygenic, there may be a threshold effect whereby the presence of disease is an all-or-none phenomenon, rather than a continuous variable.

Chromosomal abnormalities

Abnormalities in the karyotype may be either numerical or structural. Numerical abnormalities may result from failure of pairs of chromosomes to separate during meiosis (*non-disjunction*), resulting in both chromosomes being included in one nucleus, with a resulting deficiency in the other nucleus. Tetraploid cells may result from failure of separation of chromosomes so that they are all enclosed by a single nuclear membrane. Structural abnormalities result from breaking of the chromosome with irregular joining of the broken fragments. This may result in *translocation* of chromatin material from one chromosome to another, or *deletion*, with loss of chromatin material. Since genes occupy a specific place on chromosomes and groups of genes controlling certain characteristics tend to be inherited together (linked genes), it follows that abnormalities of chromosomes will result in corresponding abnormalities of genetic structure.

Sex chromosome abnormalities

Klinefelter's syndrome is characterized by a male phenotype but the individual usually possesses chromatin-positive nuclei due to an additional X chromosome giving a total of 47 chromosomes and XXY sex chromosomes. Clinically these patients have atrophic testes, infertility, eunuchoidism and mental defect.

In contrast to Klinefelter's syndrome, patients with *Turner's syndrome* are of female phenotype but are chromatin negative. The most common chromosome pattern is 45, with loss of one of the X chromosomes. These patients show sexual infantilism, webbing of the neck and cubitus valgus. There may also be other congenital defects.

Autosomal abnormalities

One of the most important is Down's syndrome (mongolism), occurring in 1 in 700 births and due to autosomal trisomy. Patients show severe mental retardation with typical physical characteristics of epicanthic folds, flat nasal bridge, protruding tongue, flattened occiput, transverse palmar crease and incurving little finger. The incidence of disease increases with advancing maternal age to 1 in 50, and this is now believed to be due to increasing risk of non-disjunction of the 21 chromosome during meiotic division to form the ovum. The syndrome can also be produced by translocation of the 21 chromosome to another chromosome, usually 15. Translocations of this pattern may be identified in a carrier mother, indicating the considerable risk of further affected children. Other autosomal trisomies are rarer but include Patau's syndrome (trisomy 13) and Edward's syndrome (trisomy 18).

Autosomal abnormalities have been detected in cells of patients with malignant disease. Polyploidy has been demonstrated in malignant cells and is one factor responsible for the hyperchromatism which is such a characteristic histological feature of malignant tumours. A chromosome with a missing arm, known as the *Philadelphia chromosome*, is a constant abnormality in chronic myeloid leukaemia. It is of interest that it is the same chromosome which is abnormal in Down's syndrome where there is an increased risk of *acute* leukaemia.

HLA system and disease

The human leucocyte antigen (HLA) system consists of a set of antigens found on the surface of lymphocytes and many other cells. There are at least four groups (A, B, C, D/Dr) and they are genetically determined, there being several alternative antigens in each group. The genes determining an individual's HLA group are found together in a region of chromosome 6 known as the major histocompatibility complex (MHC). In man, HLA groups first became important in determining the compatibility of renal allografts, rather like red cell grouping is used in blood transfusion. In the mouse it was discovered that the equivalent system was associated with some hereditary disorders and, via the immune response (Ir) genes, with the way the immune system functions. Further work in man has shown that the MHC is intimately concerned with the capacity for self–non-self recognition and with cellular co-operation in the immune response; genes controlling the level of some complement components are also found in this region. Some diseases of man have also been found to be associated with particular HLA groups. The most striking example is that of ankylosing spondylitis (a form of arthritis affecting the vertebral column) where about 90% of the patients are of HLA group B27, compared with about 9% in the general population. Nevertheless, only a minority of individuals with group B27 develop the disease, so it appears that it is not the disease itself which is inherited but the tendency to react to an environmental influence in a particular way. Several other diseases (it seems to be particularly those with immunological abnormalities) have increased frequencies of particular HLA types, e.g. Goodpasture's syndrome (D/Dr2), membranous glomerulonephritis (D/Dr3), dermatitis herpetiformis (D/Dr3) and coeliac disease (D/Dr3). A few diseases without immunological abnormalities also are linked to HLA genes, e.g. idiopathic haemochromatosis (A3) and congenital adrenal hyperplasia (B47).

Congenital malformations

These are macroscopic abnormalities of structure which are present at birth and are attributable to faulty development. Registered infant mortality from malformations has remained constant, numbering 5 per

1000 births since the beginning of the century, whereas the total infant mortality has dropped from 130 to 10.8 in 1982. The malformations, which are consequently becoming relatively more important, consist mainly of central nervous system lesions, cardiac abnormalities, hare-lip and cleft palate, defective limbs, pyloric stenosis and chromosomal abnormalities such as Down's syndrome.

Some of these abnormalities are due to genetic defects but others are a result of environmental influences within the uterus. Many of the commoner serious abnormalities, such as abnormal neural tube closure, show frequencies which suggest a *polygenic inheritance. Chromosomal abnormalities* are present in about 4% of live-born infants, but about 60% of spontaneous abortions have abnormal chromosomes. Teratogens which are known to act on the developing fetus in the uterus to produce abnormalities include irradiation, folic acid antagonists, thalidomide, some steroids and alcohol. Intrauterine *infections* which cause malformations include rubella (deafness, eye lesions, heart lesions and other central nervous system lesions) and cytomegalovirus (microgyria and neural damage).

9

Disorders of Cell Growth

Under normal circumstances, there is not much variation in the weight of organs between healthy individuals of similar age, height and weight. Cells do, however, respond to alterations in their environment and this can result in the organ decreasing or increasing in size.

Aplasia and hypoplasia

Aplasia occurs when a tissue or organ fails to develop, and *hypoplasia* occurs when they fail to reach normal size. Properly used, these terms refer to developmental abnormalities, but they are more loosely used in medicine, as for example in the term 'aplastic anaemia' (which is an acquired disorder of the bone marrow). The term *agenesis* is sometimes used to describe the developmental failure to form an organ.

Atrophy

Atrophy is the state whereby a previously normal tissue or organ becomes smaller due to a reduction in size or number of its constituent cells. Atrophy is seen particularly with nutritional deficiencies, with reduced functional activity and decreased hormone stimulus. With starvation, adipose tissue becomes reduced in amount and many organs become smaller, though this is least marked in those organs that are most vital for life—the heart and brain. Reduced functional activity causing atrophy is clearly seen in a voluntary muscle which has been paralysed. Another example is the reduced bulk of bone (*osteoporosis*) in patients confined to bed for a long time. Reduced hormonal stimulus is a potent cause of atrophy of certain organs. It occurs physiologically on such occasions as the end of lactation when the breast, which has been secreting milk, returns to its normal size. Therapeutic prednisone reduces the pituitary adrenocorticotrophic (ACTH) secretion and results in adrenal atrophy. Two special terms associated with atrophy are *fatty atrophy* and *brown atrophy*. When atrophic parenchyma is replaced with adipose tissue, the condition is called fatty atrophy: this occurs, for example, in bone marrow, lymph nodes, thymus and salivary glands. Some cells accumulate a brown pigment, lipofuscin, when they become atrophic and this is called brown atrophy. The organ, such as the heart or liver, is brown on naked-eye examination and, with the microscope, the pigment can be seen close to the nuclei. Electron microscopy shows it to be residual bodies associated with lysosomes. Atrophy implies decreased tissue bulk and usually, but not always, implies decreased cellular activity; it is important to remember that in some situations an atrophic mucosa may have an increased cell turnover, as is seen in the stomach in pernicious anaemia and the small intestine in coeliac disease.

Hypertrophy and hyperplasia

Increase in the size of an organ is usually due either to hypertrophy or to hyperplasia. These processes may occur together as a result of the same stimulus, but it is important to distinguish between them, for hyperplasia involves increased numbers of cells.

Hypertrophy is an increased bulk due to an increase in the size of the cells but not their numbers. It is most clearly seen in muscle of various types. Voluntary muscle increases in bulk with increased work, as seen when the playing arm of a tennis star is compared with his other arm. The muscle fibres of the myocardium increase in size if there is increase of resistance to the flow of blood, as seen in left ventricular hypertrophy in systemic hypertension. Similarly, the smooth muscle of the wall of the urinary bladder increases in bulk if there is obstruction to the outflow of urine.

Hyperplasia is an increased bulk due to an increase in the number of cells. There may or may not be an accompanying increase in the size of these cells. It is seen in cells which are capable of mitosis and is most often a response to cell damage or destruction or to increased hormone stimulation. The regenerating epithelium at the edge of an ulcer becomes hyperplastic if the ulcer becomes chronic. After severe haemorrhage, the red cell precursors in the bone marrow become hyperplastic and red marrow extends further into the fatty marrow. The target organs of hormones become hyperplastic when hormone levels increase. For example, the physiological hyperplasia of the thyroid at puberty and in pregnancy is caused by raised thyroid-stimulating hormone (TSH) levels, and bilateral hyperplasia of the adrenals is caused by increased ACTH levels in some forms of Cushing's syndrome.

The precise mechanisms controlling hypertrophy and hyperplasia are still unknown, but one feature that the processes have in common is that they regress once the stimulus causing them is removed.

Metaplasia

Metaplasia is the alteration which occurs when one cell type changes to another. This is quite commonly seen, most often in the epithelium of mucosal surfaces. In cigarette smokers there may be areas in the bronchial tree where the normal ciliated epithelium is replaced by squamous epithelium—*squamous metaplasia*. Squamous metaplasia can also be seen in the endocervix, the gall bladder and the urinary bladder. *Glandular metaplasia* can be seen in the urinary bladder when transitional epithelium is replaced by columnar cells. *Intestinal metaplasia* occurs in the stomach when the epithelial cells assume an intestinal pattern of mucus secretion. These changes tend to occur in epithelia subject to damage and inflammation. It must be remembered that all somatic cells contain the same genetic material but develop and function under the influence of a variety of stimuli. If these stimuli are varied, then either the structure or function of developing cells may also change and differentiate along different lines. Metaplasia also occurs in connective tissue, for example osseous metaplasia may develop in fibrous tissue.

Provided that the cells remain cytologically normal, metaplasia should be regarded as a benign, reactive, reversible condition. However, the development of nuclear atypia sometimes indicates an early stage of neoplasia.

Dysplasia

This means disordered growth and may be applied in a number of ways. Sometimes it is used to indicate maldevelopment of an organ (e.g. 'dysplastic kidney'). Another meaning is to indicate a benign proliferative disorder—as in 'benign mammary dysplasia', a synonym for fibrocystic disease of the breast. Its widest use is as a term to indicate atypia of morphology, growth and maturation of constituent cells of a tissue and it is with this meaning that it is used here. The changes are most often seen in epithelia subject to chronic low-grade damage. There may be architectural abnormalities, but the most characteristic changes are seen in the cells where there is an increased nuclear : cytoplasmic ratio, increased nuclear staining and sometimes irregularity of the nucleus. These changes occur as a result of many stimuli including infection, trauma, cytotoxic drugs and irradiation, and may be superimposed on hyperplasia or metaplasia. It takes much skill and is sometimes impossible to distinguish reversible lesions from those which are likely to progress to the development of a tumour.

10

Neoplasia

The development of a neoplasm (a term synonymous with tumour or new growth) is due to another disorder of cell growth. The process is similar to hyperplasia in that there is an increase in cell numbers, but differs in that the proliferation becomes uncontrolled. It is not easy to find a definition of a neoplasm to which there are no objections. The classical one is that of Rupert Willis who wrote that a neoplasm is 'an abnormal mass of tissue, the growth of which exceeds and is uncoordinated with that of the normal tissue and persists in the same excessive manner after cessation of the stimuli which caused its growth'. A shorter definition is that neoplasia is that form of hyperplasia in which the new cells transmit the abnormal proliferative capacity to their offspring, independently of the initiating stimulus. These definitions are derived from observations of experimental chemical carcinogenesis and are difficult to apply to many human tumours, where we often do not know the nature of the initiating stimuli and therefore cannot know whether they are still present. When a cause is known, however, as with aromatic amines and carcinoma of the urinary bladder, or cigarette smoking and carcinoma of the bronchus, it is apparent that once the neoplasm has developed, the removal of the stimulus does not cause regression. Indeed, in the case of tumours of the bladder, the exposure to the chemical may have been very many years before the appearance of the tumour. These observations fit in with the concept implicit in the definition, which is that the tumour cells have to some extent become autonomous and are not subject to the same controls as normal cells. Their growth may still be influenced by many factors, such as hormonal environment or oxygen supply, but they are free from some of the normal controls.

There are many different kinds of neoplasm. They vary from small, slowly growing nodules which have virtually no effect on the individual, to rapidly enlarging, quickly spreading tumours that kill in a short time. Systems of classification have therefore been developed to help diagnosis, prognosis and treatment as well as to assist understanding of their nature. The most useful characteristics of an individual tumour to be aware of are: (a) whether it is benign or malignant, (b) its site of origin, and (c) its cell type. If it is malignant, one needs to know how far it has spread (its stage) and how poorly differentiated it is (its grade).

Features of benign and malignant neoplasm (Table 2)

Most tumours seen clinically can be easily characterized as benign or malignant after microscopic examination. The concept of malignancy is that of a tumour which, left to itself, invades neighbouring tissue, spreads to distant sites (metastasizes) and kills the patient. On the other

Table 2. Typical features of benign and malignant neoplasms.*

		Benign	*Malignant*
Behaviour	Growth rate	Slow	Fast
	Expansion	Yes	Yes
	Invasion	No	Yes
	Metastasis	No	Yes
	Cessation of growth	Frequent	Rare
Naked-eye appearance	Demarcation	Good	Poor
	Margins	Sharp (capsule often)	Irregular (capsule rare)
	Cut surface	Smooth	Irregular
	Necrosis	Uncommon	Frequent
Histological appearance	Architecture	Similar to normal	Often lost
	Differentiation	Good	Poor
	Invasion	Absent	Present
	Mitotic rate	Low	Increased
Cytological appearance	Differentiation	Good	Bad
	Nuclear–cytoplasmic ratio	Low	High
	Nuclear outline	Smooth	Irregular
	Hyperchromatic	No	Yes
	Pleomorphism	No	Yes
	Nucleoli	Normal	Increased
	Aneuploidy	No	Yes

*The two most important features of malignancy are invasion and metastasis.

hand, a typical benign tumour grows slowly, does not infiltrate or metastasize and, if it harms the patient, does so by an incidental complication such as haemorrhage or obstruction of a hollow viscus. Typical features of benign and malignant neoplasms have come to be recognized both in behaviour and in morphological appearances. Indeed, the morphological features, particularly the histology and cytology, are the best predictors of biological behaviour. It must be remembered, however, that benign and malignant are ends of a spectrum and between them are varying shades. There are exceptions to all of the typical features which characterize the two behaviour patterns. These features are discussed below, with some of the exceptions.

Behaviour

A benign tumour typically grows slowly by expansion. It enlarges rather like a balloon and compresses surrounding tissue. It does not send out processes into surrounding tissue or metastasize, and often there is spontaneous cessation of growth. Exceptions include: keratoacanthoma (a benign squamous cell tumour of the skin) which grows rapidly and infiltrates but resolves; pleomorphic adenoma (a benign tumour of the salivary gland) which may also have an infiltrative growth pattern.

The typical malignant lesion grows fast and, in addition to expanding, it sends out processes into surrounding tissue to infiltrate them. The term 'cancer' is widely used for malignant tumours because of the resemblance of the prongs to the legs and claws of the crab. Frequently, cells become detached and travel in channels such as veins and lymphatics to settle and grow in other organs; the original tumour is known as the *primary*, the metastatic deposits are often called *secondaries*. It is only very rarely that established malignant tumours spontaneously regress, but there are well-documented cases, some of which appear to be due to an immunological reaction to the tumour. Success rate in treating malignant tumours is often measured as the percentage five-year survival of patients, but with some of the more slowly growing tumours, such as well-differentiated papillary carcinoma of the thyroid, it is necessary to talk in terms of 20-year survival figures, or even longer. Basal cell carcinoma of the skin is a tumour which infiltrates but does not metastasize.

Naked-eye appearances

The typical naked-eye appearances of a benign tumour, such as a fibroadenoma of the breast, are a reflection of its growth pattern. It tends to be round, well demarcated from surrounding normal tissue, sometimes with a capsule formed from compressed normal tissue. Its cut surface is smooth and, because it is expanding, often bulges outwards, appearing convex. Necrosis is uncommon but can occur especially if blood vessels are compressed. Malignant tumours tend to be poorly demarcated, as you would expect from their infiltrative tendency; their margins are usually irregular and a capsule is rare. The cut surface is sometimes convex but can be concave, as in scirrhous carcinoma of the breast where there is a marked fibrous reaction to the tumour. Necrosis is more commonly seen in malignant tumours. Naked-eye appearances are only a guide because non-neoplastic lesions can stimulate malignancy.

Histological appearances

The architecture of a benign tumour tends to be similar to that of the parent tissue and the cells closely resemble the parent cells, forming glands or ducts or making keratin, depending on their type; invasion is absent. Interestingly, pleomorphic adenoma of the salivary gland is an exception to all these rules, but it is benign. The mitotic rate is usually low in benign tumours. In malignancy, the cells often fail to differentiate fully so that the architectural relationships are lost, differentiated structures are not properly formed and invasion is demonstrable. Some tumours lack all features of differentiation and these are described as *anaplastic*. Mitoses are often prominent and some of them may be abnormal. Some well-differentiated malignant tumours lack these features; follicular carcinoma of the thyroid is a good example where vascular invasion may be the only indicator of malignant behaviour.

Cytological appearances

These are the features of individual cells, either as part of a histological section or as isolated cells prepared from smears or imprints. Cells from a benign tumour tend to resemble the normal cells of the tissue. They are therefore well differentiated, have a normal nuclear–cytoplasmic ratio and their nuclear outline is smooth. The cells have a normal amount of nucleoprotein and stain normally with nuclear stains; also there is not much variation between cells. The nuclei have a normal complement of chromosomes (they are euploid). Malignant cells tend not to mature properly; they are therefore less well differentiated. Some changes are seen in the cytoplasm but the most important indicators of malignancy are seen in the nucleus. The nuclei tend to be larger, giving an increased nuclear–cytoplasmic ratio. The nuclear outline tends to be irregular and the nucleus takes up more stain, i.e. it is hyperchromatic, often showing coarsely clumped chromatin. If different cells are compared, they can be seen to vary in size and shape more than normal—that is, they are pleomorphic. Nucleoli are often more prominent in malignant cells. If chromosomes are studied, malignant tumours often show populations of cells with abnormal numbers of chromosomes—aneuploidy.

Nomenclature and classification of neoplasms

No nomenclature of neoplasms is universally accepted because no system has yet been devised which is completely satisfactory. Various systems have been proposed, of which the *histogenetic* classification is most widely used. This is based on the cell type from which the tumour arises. The division into *behaviour* patterns of benign and malignant forms has already been discussed. The *shape* of a tumour is sometimes used in classification because, for some tumours, prognosis depends partly on the pattern of tumour growth, whether it is a solid plaque or frond-like outgrowths (e.g. urinary bladder tumours). The *site of origin* is clearly important and it is necessary to combine this information with a histogenetic classification, for tumours occurring in a particular organ may arise from different cell types. Classification based on the *embryological origin* of the tissue is of limited value and, at the moment, so is that based on *aetiology*.

The terminology followed here is based largely on histogenesis. Willis grouped tumours into five major groups; four of them depend on whether their origin was from epithelium, connective tissue, the haemolymphohistiocytic tissue or the nervous system. The fifth miscellaneous group includes certain tumours which were difficult to fit in with others. With each major group, there are tumours arising from different cell types and for each cell type there may be a benign or malignant version. There are so many different types of tumour that it is difficult to make generalizations, but there is some virtue in looking at outlines of the major groups before learning the greater detail in systemic pathology.

Epithelial neoplasms

Descriptive terms indicating *shape* are frequently used as part of the designation of these tumours, but it must be remembered that when used on their own, these words may simply indicate the form of a lesion, which is not necessarily even neoplastic. A *polyp* is a pedunculated mass arising from an epithelial surface. A *papilloma* indicates frond-like outgrowths arising from an epithelial surface. An *annular* mass is one which encircles the lumen of a hollow viscus. Other descriptive terms describe the *consistency* of a mass. A *scirrhous* tumour is a hard mass, the hardness being due to the marked fibroblastic (desmoplastic) reaction produced by some carcinomas, particularly in the breast. When there is no fibrous reaction and the mass consists of masses of malignant cells, the consistency may be soft like brain and the word *encephaloid* is sometimes used. If a tumour produces large amounts of mucin, it may be called a *colloid* tumour. Though these words describing consistency are widely used, they have not proved very useful in classification and it is better to characterize the lesions by histology.

Benign epithelial neoplasms

These have names which often describe their cell type and their shape. *Squamous cell papillomas* are composed of cells similar to those found in the prickle cell layer of the skin and are commonly found on skin surfaces, where they are often called warts. Many of these are due to virus infection and will disappear when the virus is no longer active. This illustrates how difficult it may be to distinguish hyperplasia from a true benign tumour. Some benign tumours of squamous cells are called *acanthomas*. Some benign tumours of the skin in elderly people are composed of cells resembling the basal cells of the skin and these are called *basal cell papillomas* (seborrhoeic warts). Transitional cell papillomas may occur in the urothelial tract, but most papillary lesions in this site are carcinomas. *Adenomas* are benign tumours of secretory or duct-type epithelium. They may project from an epithelial surface or grow in the substance of glandular tissue. Sometimes adenomas are largely cystic in their make-up, with papillary projections into their cavity. A good example of this type is the papillary serous cystadenoma of the ovary.

Malignant epithelial tumours

These are called *carcinomas* and are subdivided according to cell type.

Squamous cell carcinomas, sometimes called epitheliomas, are composed of cells resembling those of the prickle cell layer of the skin; they develop intercellular bridges (prickles) visible with the light microscope and may produce keratin. Because of the disordered cell growth invading surrounding tissues, this keratin may not be on the surface and can be in the middle of cell nests, forming keratin pearls. These tumours arise at sites normally lined by stratified squamous epithelium, for example the skin, lips, buccal cavity, pharynx, oesophagus, larynx and cervix uteri. They also develop as a result of metaplasia in sites normally lined by epithelium of another type; this tends to occur when glandular epithelium has been subject to chronic irritation resulting in squamous metaplasia. The best example of this is in the bronchus where squamous carcinoma is the commonest type. It also occurs, though less commonly, in the urinary tract and gall bladder. Squamous carcinomas are invasive and show a tendency for lymphatic spread to occur before blood spread.

Basal cell carcinomas occur on the skin and infiltrate locally but do not metastasize.

Transitional cell carcinomas occur most commonly in the urinary bladder but can be seen anywhere in the urothelial tract. They tend to grow in papillary or solid, plaque-like forms. The diagnosis of carcinoma is made here even without seeing invasion; papillary lesions only have to show a mild degree of hyperplastic thickening or cellular atypia and the label carcinoma is put on them. This is because they show such a great tendency to recur and infiltrate that the threshold for diagnosing malignancy is lower than elsewhere. It is interesting to compare the situation with that of adenomatous polyps in the large bowel, where striking cellular proliferation and gross cellular atypia are seen but where carcinoma is not normally diagnosed until there is invasion through the muscularis mucosae. It is another example of tumour pathology having general rules which are very considerably altered in specific instances. Transitional cell tumours tend to recur and infiltrate locally and to metastasize late, via lymphatics and the bloodstream.

Adenocarcinomas arise from secretory or ductular epithelium in many organs. The gastrointestinal tract with the pancreas, biliary tree and liver account for the largest number of primaries, but these also occur in other organs such as the breast, kidney, ovary, prostate and thyroid.

Most adenocarcinomas arise from glandular surface epithelium or secretory glands. They tend to metastasize first by way of lymphatics and later by the bloodstream. Others, such as adenocarcinoma of the kidney, more often spread via the bloodstream.

Undifferentiated (anaplastic) carcinomas are those which lack features, such as keratin or glands, which enable them to be positively identified. They are usually the more malignant versions of the better differentiated tumours and do not constitute a distinct entity.

The number of tumours which can be positively identified increases if special techniques are used. A reticulin preparation usually shows a carcinoma growing in packets, whereas sarcomas lack this feature. Histochemistry can show, for example, the presence of epithelial mucin in the cells of an apparently undifferentiated tumour, revealing it as an adenocarcinoma. Immunohistochemistry can reveal substances, such as prostatic acid phosphatase, which can indicate the type of tumour and also the likely primary site. Electron microscopy can show up organelles, such as melanosomes, which can indicate the nature of a tumour. Nevertheless, we are still left with many carcinomas which are not identified and some tumours which are so poorly differentiated that we cannot even tell whether they are carcinomas or other tumours such as sarcomas or lymphomas. These are usually very aggressive tumours with a poor prognosis.

Tumours of connective tissue, muscle and vessels

Although it is convenient to think of connective tissue cells as being of a specific type, such as fibroblasts or cartilage cells, it seems that these cells can be induced to form different types of matrix. For this reason different kinds of tissue can often be seen in one tumour in this group. It is customary to classify these tumours according to the predominant tumour cell or the most malignant component. An important example is when malignant tumour cells are forming osteoid, the protein matrix of bone. Experience has shown that this feature indicates the aggressive behaviour of an osteosarcoma whatever the other elements are forming.

The names given to the benign tumours in this group of non-haemo-poietic mesenchyme consist of the suffix 'oma' combined with the prefix indicating cell of origin. The malignant tumours are called sarcomas, with similar prefixes to their benign counterparts. Sarcomas are more inclined to spread via the bloodstream than are carcinomas. The undifferentiated sarcomas are usually described according to the shape of the predominant cell, e.g. spindle-cell, round-cell or polygonal cell sarcoma, but this is not particularly useful. Examples are listed in Table

Table 3. Examples of benign and malignant tumours of connective tissue, muscle and vessels.

	Benign	*Malignant*
Fibrous tissue	Fibroma	Fibrosarcoma
Adipose tissue	Lipoma	Liposarcoma
Bone	Osteoma	Osteosarcoma
Cartilage	Chondroma	Chondrosarcoma
Smooth muscle	Leiomyoma	Leiomyosarcoma
Striated muscle	Rhabdomyoma	Rhabdomyosarcoma
Blood vessels		Haemangiosarcoma
Lymphatics		Lymphangiosarcoma
Synovium	Benign synovioma	Synovial sarcoma
Mesothelium	Benign mesothelioma	Mesothelioma

3 and more information is given in the systemic pathology section. It will be noticed from this table that haemangioma and lymphangioma have not been included in the list of benign tumours. This is because they more commonly fall into the category of malformation than benign tumour as defined on p. 68.

Neoplasms of the haemopoietic and lymphohistiocytic systems

This group is unusual in that true benign tumours do not occur in it, though some premalignant lesions are recognized. The malignant tumours are mainly leukaemias and lymphomas. The leukaemias predominantly affect the blood and bone marrow and are widely disseminated at an early stage. The lymphomas are particularly found in tissue with concentrations of lymphocytes, especially lymph nodes and the spleen. Although they can be widely disseminated early, they often present as a localized tumour mass. They are discussed further under systemic pathology (see p. 221).

Neoplasms of the nervous system

These are derived either from the nerve cells themselves or from the supporting elements. Tumours of the neurons are very rare in the adult for these are normally post-mitotic cells. Some tumours of childhood, such as the medulloblastoma (central nervous system) or neuroblastoma (adrenal medulla and sympathetic chain), may contain neoplastic nerve cells. A more mature version is the ganglioneuroma. Within the central nervous system, the main tumours of the supporting elements are the gliomas (astrocytoma, oligodendroglioma and ependymoma). These are malignant tumours but their effect may depend more on their site than on their intrinsic invasiveness. An interesting feature of their behaviour is that though they may metastasize within the central nervous system, they do not naturally metastasize outside it. The supporting cells of the cranial and peripheral nerves are the Schwann cells and these give rise to nerve sheath tumours, neurofibromas and neurilemmomas (schwannomas). These are benign lesions but occasionally a neurofibrosarcoma can develop. The so-called 'acoustic neuroma' of the VIIIth nerve is a schwannoma. Meningiomas probably develop from the arachnoid granulations; they are benign tumours but can be locally invasive.

Miscellaneous neoplasms

Malignant melanoma

This is a highly malignant tumour which arises from melanocytes (the pigment forming cells found in the epidermis). Though the tumours tend to present in the skin, the cells are probably neural crest derived and this gives them some characteristics which make them different from epithelial cells.

Teratomas

These are tumours of totipotential cells—that is, of cells which can differentiate into tissue of all three germ layers and sometimes with trophoblastic and yolk sac elements as well. It is not always possible to see cells of all three layers and, indeed, the more malignant the tumour, the less easy it is to demonstrate all the elements. These tumours usually arise from the germ cells in the gonads but can develop in extragonadal sites, particularly in the midline. It is interesting that teratomas exhibit different behaviour in the male and female. Almost all teratomas in the ovary are benign (dermoid cyst—benign cystic teratoma), but almost all those in the testis are malignant.

It is important not to confuse the word 'hamartoma' with 'teratoma'. A *hamartoma* is a benign tumour-like malformation which consists of tissue normally found at that site but is present in the wrong amount. These lesions usually, but not always, grow with the individual and stop when the individual stops growing.

Choriocarcinoma

This is a word used for a malignant tumour which shows trophoblastic differentiation. It is applied to two different types of lesion: one is the teratoma which has trophoblastic elements, the other is a tumour found in the uterus and derived from the trophoblast of the placenta. This second type is very unusual in that it is a tumour of 'non-self' which is not rejected by the individual's immune system.

Blastomas

These are uncommon tumours which occur most often in childhood where they are malignant, consisting of immature tissue. Neuroblastomas (adrenal medulla) and nephroblastoma (kidney—Wilms' tumour) are the commonest, but blastomas also occur in the brain (medulloblastoma), eye (retinoblastoma) and liver (hepatoblastoma). There are similarities in their histological appearances and the bulk of them consists of sheets of small undifferentiated cells with little cytoplasm. Some of them show attempts at differentiation: the nephroblastoma, for example, often shows primitive glomeruli and tubules. Those occurring outside the central nervous system may metastasize via the bloodstream. Unfortunately the term 'blastoma' is also applied to some benign tumours which may occur in adults (osteoblastoma in bone; haemangioblastoma in the cerebellum).

Staging and grading of malignant neoplasms

There are many different types of malignant neoplasm, showing a wide range of behaviour. Even for a tumour of a particular cell type, for example adenocarcinoma of the large bowel or transitional cell carcinoma of the bladder, there is considerable variation in outlook (prognosis) for the patient. Two further pieces of information help to give a better assessment of the likely behaviour of a tumour in an individual patient. One of these is to know how far the tumour has spread at the time of diagnosis (*staging*), and the other is to know how poorly differentiated it is (*grading*).

Clearly a patient with a large tumour mass in the colon and metastases in the liver and brain has a different prognosis from one who has had a small polyp removed which showed superficial invasion through the muscularis mucosae, though the diagnosis in both might be adenocarcinoma of the colon. Cuthbert Dukes showed that by identifying the extent of spread of rectal carcinoma in surgically removed specimens, he could give a good assessment of the likely five-year survival of the patient. He found that the important stages were invasion into the muscle coat but not through the bowel wall (A), through the bowel wall but not into lymph nodes (B), and with lymph node involvement (C). The approximate five-year survivals are: A, 80%; B, 60%; and C, 30%. Similar systems have been evolved for tumours in other sites. These are systems of pathological staging but one of their disadvantages is that they are not applicable to tumours which are not widely excised. Therefore, clinical systems have been evolved and are particularly used for tumours which are treated by radiotherapy and chemotherapy. It is important to remember that staging systems are only comparable if they use the same methods and the same criteria. For example, clinical staging of a breast carcinoma is altered by the presence of palpable axillary lymph nodes. Pathological staging of the specimen might show that these nodes were reactive and not involved by tumour. In another patient, pathological examination might reveal small lymph node deposits that were not palpable clinically. Most staging systems are based on features of the primary tumour (particularly size), the presence of lymph node deposits, and whether or not there are distant metastases. Many systems have been drawn up but the most widely used is the TNM system (tumour, node, metastasis) which the World Health Organisation has adopted to make studies from different centres comparable. Points are given for various features and a tumour finishes up with a numerical score. Staging tumours accurately is a detailed and time-consuming exercise but when properly used the information obtained is valuable.

Assessing the degree of differentiation of tumour cells (grading) is a pathological exercise. It has been shown in many situations (e.g. transitional cell carcinoma of the urinary bladder, teratoma of the testis) that for a given stage of spread, the prognosis is affected by how poorly differentiated the tumour cells are: the poorer the differentiation, the worse the prognosis. Malignant tumours are usually reported as being well, moderately or poorly differentiated, though some numerical schemes have been introduced.

There are difficulties in making grading reproducible. One is that tumours may vary considerably in differentiation in different areas: in general, the most poorly differentiated area is taken. Another is that there is variation in the criteria used to assess differentiation: this can be avoided by drawing up criteria which are as objective as possible.

The terms staging and grading are often confused, possibly because poorly differentiated tumours tend to have spread further at the time of diagnosis. They are both attempts at assessing tumours but they are quite different exercises.

The effects of neoplasms

Tumours can produce many different symptoms and signs. Even a large destructive mass is not necessarily neoplastic, for other pathological processes such as inflammation have to be considered.

Benign tumours

Benign tumours grow locally by expansion and so they usually appear simply as a mass or with pressure effects. The latter are commoner when the tumour is growing in a confined space, for example the cranial cavity where raised intracranial pressure can develop compressing the brain including its vital centres. Another way in which serious effects occasionally occur is when a tumour on a stalk undergoes torsion which then results in venous congestion and haemorrhage or venous infarction.

Benign tumours can produce distant effects by secreting hormones. This is seen with adenomas of the endocrine glands, for example a basophil adenoma of the pituitary can produce ACTH, causing bilateral adrenal hyperplasia and Cushing's syndrome.

Malignant tumours

Malignant tumours grow by expansion and infiltration and also metastasize. They therefore cause symptoms and signs via the primary growth and the secondary deposits but also have systemic effects.

Local growth

This produces similar *pressure effects* as do benign tumours but they are usually more marked because of the faster growth rate. There is frequently *impairment of function* of an organ in which a tumour arises. *Ulceration* is common when a tumour arises on an epithelial surface; *perforation* can follow, as with carcinoma of the colon. *Fistula* formation may develop when the tumour penetrates through to another epithelial surface, for example between the stomach and the transverse colon—a gastrocolic fistula. When the lumen of a viscus is narrowed, *obstruction* to flow of its contents can occur, as with intestinal obstruction from carcinoma of the colon, or hydronephrosis developing from carcinoma of the ureter. *Invasion of nerves* can produce effects at a distance from the tumour. An example is carcinoma of the apex of the lung (Pancoast's tumour) which invades the neck; involvement of the brachial plexus gives symptoms and signs in the arm, while involvement of the sympathetic chain gives ptosis, enophthalmos and reduction of sweating on that side of the face (Horner's syndrome). *Bleeding* is a common complication; it can be low grade and, if it occurs into the gastrointestinal tract, may not be suspected until the patient presents with iron deficiency anaemia. It may also be massive if a large vessel is invaded. *Destruction of vital structures*, particularly those in the midline of the brainstem, will produce death at an early stage, even with a small tumour.

Metastasis

Spread to distant sites is a characteristic of malignant tumours. The loss of adhesion allows the cells to break off and to travel along natural channels, particularly lymphatic and blood vessels but also across serous cavities. It is extremely uncommon for tumours to seed along the lumen of a mucosal surface, unless there has been surgical interference causing a breach in the mucosa. The factors which influence the development of metastases are still largely unknown, though it is clear that local factors are important because secondary tumours form more commonly in some organs than others. Evidence, largely based on a study of the spread of malignant melanomas of the skin, has accumulated which indicates that an immune reaction to the tumour may develop and this can limit the primary tumour and restrict the growth of metastases. The cellular reaction around many malignant tumours may have a similar role. Rapidly growing melanomas indicate a deficiency of the host immune reaction.

1. *Lymphatic spread.* Tumour cells have the property of being able to infiltrate through the thin-walled lymphatic channels in their neighbourhood, and then grow along the lymphatics (permeation) or be carried along by the lymph to the lymph nodes into which the lymphatics drain. Microscopically, the first evidence that tumour cells have arrived in a lymph node is the appearance of a small clump at the periphery in the cortical sinus. If the tumour cells are able to continue to grow, they usually do so, within the sinuses at first, but eventually they will completely replace all the lymphoid tissue of the node, and even extend beyond the confines of the capsule of the node. The lymph nodes in this way temporarily hold up the progress of the malignant tumour, and this is the basis for one of the standard surgical treatments of malignant disease—block dissection of the regional lymph nodes. However, the malignant cells frequently pass on from one lymph node to another and it is not an uncommon clinical experience to find a metastasis in a lymph node which is remote from the site of origin. Sometimes neoplastic cells will spread along lymph channels in retrograde fashion because the normal drainage area has been blocked by the formation of lymph node metastases. This is one explanation for metastases being observed in unexpected places. The malignant cells may find their way eventually into the thoracic duct and thus be disseminated widely in the lungs and the rest of the body by way of the bloodstream. Tumour may also spread by way of perineural spaces, which is quite a frequent phenomenon, and is probably the cause of the development of pain in many instances.

2. *Bloodstream spread.* The arterial wall is relatively resistant to infiltration by malignant neoplasms, which gain access to the bloodstream more frequently by way of veins or capillaries. When tumour cells penetrate through the endothelial lining of these vessels, they are liable to become the nidus for thrombus formation, and fragmentation of these malignant thrombi is the starting point of some of the bloodborne metastases; free circulation of individual malignant cells also occurs. The malignant cells are carried in the venous system either through the right side of the heart to the lung capillaries or, if they start within the alimentary tract, through the portal vein to the sinusoids of the liver. Most of these tumour emboli die at their point of impact, some proliferate to form metastases, others permeate along the capillary walls to reach wider channels distally, whence they disseminate. In the case of

the lungs, this is by way of the systemic arteries and so to all parts of the body; in the case of the liver, it will first be into the hepatic vein and the inferior vena cava and thence through the right side of the heart to the lungs.

3. *Transcoelomic spread*. Once a malignant tumour has infiltrated through the endothelial surface of the serous cavities of the body, it is liable to appear in the form of secondary nodules elsewhere in that cavity. These nodules may be few in number or be so numerous as to form a practically continuous lining over the membrane surface. It is considered by most that this 'transcoelomic' spread occurs because tumour cells fragment from their site of original penetration into the cavity and subsequently seed themselves elsewhere on the membrane surface. There are some, however, who consider that spread by way of the lymphatic network beneath the membrane surface plays an important part in the dissemination of the tumour. This development of secondary tumours in the walls of serous cavities is quite a common event, especially within the peritoneum and the pleural cavity. The tumours usually lead to the formation of fluid exudates, and the cytological identification of malignant cells in the aspirated fluid is helpful in diagnosis.

The effects of metastases are similar to those of primary tumours at the same site. Indeed, when a tumour presents in a particular organ it is always sensible to consider whether it could be a secondary from elsewhere. Most intracranial neoplasms in the elderly are secondaries; similarly, most circumscribed malignant deposits in bone are metastases.

Non-metastatic systemic effects

Malignant tumours often have effects on parts of the body other than where they are growing. These can be general and ill-defined or may be localized to particular organs.

1. *Cancer cachexia* is a syndrome characterized by anorexia, weight loss, weakness, pallor and anaemia. This is often seen with advanced malignancy and there are probably many factors playing a part in its development, only some of them known. Deficient food intake is important, but in addition the presence of the tumour means that the patient does not respond normally to this starvation.

2. Examples of *non-metastatic syndromes* associated with neoplasms are found in every organ system. Some of them are rare, but collectively they are seen in appreciable numbers of cancer patients.

Many different skin lesions can be seen, for example *dermatomyositis* which is a form of inflammation in the skin and muscles. About half the patients over the age of 40 with this disorder have an internal malignancy. The presence of *anaemia* is easily understood after bleeding or when the marrow is replaced by tumour, but these are not the only reasons for its occurrence. There is often a toxic depression of the marrow and sometimes, especially with lymphomas, a haemolytic anaemia. Red cell *polycythaemia* can occur particularly with adenocarcinoma of the kidney. *Thrombophlebitis migrans* (fleeting thrombosis of superficial veins) was originally described with carcinoma of the pancreas but can occur with other tumours. *Finger clubbing* is commonly seen with internal malignancies, and subperiosteal new bone formation in the tibia, fibula, radius and ulna (hypertrophic pulmonary osteoarthropathy) is sometimes seen with carcinoma of the bronchus. Degenerative lesions of the central nervous system occur without metastases. A good example is *cerebellar degeneration* with carcinoma of the bronchus. Endocrine effects can be due either to endocrine tumours producing their normal hormones (eutopic) or to tumours producing hormones not normally associated with that cell type (ectopic hormone production). Examples of the latter are *ACTH* and *parathormone* produced by carcinoma of the bronchus.

The explanation of most of these effects remains unknown. Polycythaemia and renal adenocarcinoma are linked by the production of erythropoietin. Eutopic hormone production is easy to understand; ectopic hormone production is probably a function of disordered protein synthesis of the malignant cells. In some cases it is believed that an immunological reaction plays a part. Dermatomyositis has some features of an immune complex disorder.

Some polypeptide molecules produced by tumours can be detected in the serum or on the cells. A few of these, called *tumour markers*, are useful in diagnosis or in monitoring treatment. High levels of human chorionic gonadotrophin (HCG) occur in the serum with trophoblastic tumours. Alpha-fetoprotein (AFP) is a marker of hepatoma, a malignant tumour of hepatocytes and some malignant teratomas. Carcinoembryonic antigen (CEA) occurs particularly with tumours of the gastrointestinal tract. Prostatic acid phosphatase can be present in the serum of patients with prostatic carcinoma, as well as being demonstrable in the tumour cells. It is important to remember that these molecules are not really specific for malignancy but can be useful in diagnosis and follow-up if interpreted correctly.

The causes of malignant tumours

There is no single cause of cancer. There are many different cancers and the origin of each is multifactorial. At the moment we are only partially able to understand the mechanisms of development of a few tumours. Many aetiological factors have, however, been identified, and these can be divided into hereditary and environmental groups.

Heredity

For some tumours, hereditary factors are strong. Polyposis coli is inherited as a Mendelian dominant which results in multiple adenomas of the large bowel leading to the development of carcinoma. Retinoblastoma, a childhood tumour of the eye, may be sporadic but when familial it is inherited as a Mendelian dominant. Another inherited condition is xeroderma pigmentosa in which squamous carcinomas and other neoplasms develop in the skin of sun-exposed areas. In this condition it is not the tumours which are inherited but the inability to repair DNA after it has been damaged by irradiation. The persistent altered DNA then results in malignancy.

For common malignancies there does not seem to be a very strong familial incidence. Some families do have a higher incidence of particular tumours, for example carcinoma of the breast is commoner in first-degree relatives of patients than would be expected by chance. Polygenic inheritance of a tendency to develop this tumour is one explanation, but it is difficult to exclude shared environmental factors.

With some chromosomal abnormalities, particularly Down's syndrome, there is a higher incidence of leukaemia.

Environment

Environmental factors which have been shown to influence the development of cancer are: (1) chemicals, (2) ionizing radiations, and (3) some chronic infections. If the internal environment is considered, then one can add some non-infectious chronic inflammations and hormonal influences.

Chemical carcinogens

The first indication that chemical carcinogens existed came from industry. Scrotal cancer was shown to develop in chimney sweeps; cancer of the skin of hands, arms and scrotum appeared in workers in shale-oil extraction distilleries and the mule-spinners of cotton mills; and cancer of the bladder was a risk among those working in the rubber and plastics industry and handling aniline dyes. It has also been shown that there is an increased incidence of cancer of the lung and other tumours among cigarette smokers. Experimental verification of the existence of specific chemical carcinogens first came in 1915 when Japanese workers produced cancers in the ears of rabbits which they had painted for many months with tar solutions. Since then a number of other chemical carcinogens have been identified and these fall into three main groups. The first consists of polycyclic aromatic hydrocarbons, which are responsible for the oil, soot, and tar tumours of humans, notably 3,4 benzpyrene. They produce tumours in animals at the site of application or injection. The second group consists of the aromatic amines, which can induce bladder tumours in man. Benzidene and β-naphthylamine are potent members of the group. β-naphthylamine also produces similar tumours in dogs, but other species are less susceptible. The amines produce tumours at a distance from the site of application, and their carcinogenic effect depends on their conversion to orthohydroxyamines in the body. The third group of chemical carcinogens comprise the azo-compounds increasingly used in industry to colour food. Members of the group, a well-known example being 'butter-yellow' (para-dimethylamino-azo-benzene), produce carcinoma of the liver when fed to rats. These therefore are similar to the aromatic amines in that they act at a distance from their site of application.

Ionizing radiations

Skin surfaces, especially of fair-haired people, when exposed for long periods to bright sunlight, are liable to develop keratoses (precancerous lesions), some of which, if untreated, sooner or later progress to frank squamous cell carcinoma. In the early years after the discovery of x-rays and radium, workers in the field subjected themselves to undue exposure to these radiations, developed radiation burns as a consequence, and many years later a number suffered from carcinoma of the exposed skin. Excessive unscreened irradiation was also used at one time for treatment of diseases of the thyroid gland and this led subsequently to the development of malignant tumours of the thyroid gland, pharynx or larynx. The incidence of such tumours is now negligible because of adequate protective measures. Radium salts, if ingested, find their way to bones and may precipitate tumour formation. For example, a number of cases of bone sarcoma occurred among factory girls who had been applying luminous paint containing radium to watch dials for some years. They had absorbed the radium by pointing the brushes between their lips. A high incidence of carcinoma, especially of the bronchus, has been shown to exist among the underground workers in the Schneeberg mines in Saxony and the Joachimsthal mines in Czechoslovakia, in both of which the mined ores are radioactive. Carcinoma of the liver has developed in man after intravenous injection of thorotrast (thorium dioxide), used at one time as a contrast medium in radiology. The injected thorotrast was taken up in the reticuloendothelial (Kupffer) cells in the liver. Carcinoma of thyroid has occurred in some young people whose thymus had been irradiated in infancy. Leukaemia has developed with much increased frequency among the Japanese who were exposed to atom bombs at Hiroshima and Nagasaki. The leukaemia arose earlier in those who had relatively the greater exposure. Radiologists have been shown to have a higher incidence of leukaemia than other physicians. There has been an increased incidence of leukaemia among those cases of ankylosing spondylitis submitted to radiotherapy and it is claimed that leukaemia is commoner in children whose mothers have had diagnostic x-ray pelvimetry during their pregnancy than in those who have not been so exposed.

In those instances where malignant disease has developed at sites of previous irradiation damage, it is reasonable to assume that the radiations were the cause of the cancer. On those occasions when this tissue damage has not been apparent following irradiation, the significance of radiation being carcinogenic in any given situation has been assessed on a statistical basis. In the examples quoted above, the relationship has proved to be highly significant.

Chronic inflammation

Some chronic infections and also some non-infective chronic inflammatory conditions are associated with the development of neoplasia. Squamous carcinoma developing in the skin at the edge of a discharging sinus from chronic osteomyelitis was one of the first to be noticed. It was called *Marjolin's ulcer*. Now that chronic osteomyelitis is rare it is not seen, but a similar neoplasm arises in the edge of chronic venous stasis ulcers. The parasitic infection *Schistosomiasis* produces chronic inflammation in several sites, including the urinary bladder where it appears to be responsible for the development of squamous carcinoma.

Not many infections have a well-documented carcinogenic effect but if animal models of disease are considered, then viruses clearly cause tumours. This was first shown by Rous who, in 1911, transferred a sarcoma of the pectoral muscle of a Plymouth Rock fowl to others of the same breed by means of a cell-free filtrate. In 1922, Shope induced a skin papilloma in wild cotton-tail rabbits. Other conditions, especially leukaemias and other forms of lymphoid neoplasms, have been described and viruses have been identified as the causative agents. Knowing that viruses can enter nuclei and become involved with replicating molecules, it is perhaps not surprising that proliferation of the host cell is sometimes induced and that this can become neoplastic. In human neoplasms, however, the search for causative viruses has not been as successful as anticipated. Certainly host cell proliferation can be induced and tumour-like conditions appear (probably the best example is that of the verruca vulgaris, common wart), but as yet no human cancer has been proved to be due to a virus. The best evidence for virus involvement is in Burkitt's lymphoma, a malignant tumour found particularly in children in Africa. There is a strong association with the EB (Epstein–Barr) virus, which causes glandular fever in temperate regions, and with malaria. Circumstantial evidence suggests that EB virus infection early in life combined with some other factor, such as malaria, which changes the host immunity, results in neoplasia. Nasopharyngeal carcinoma in some areas of the world is also associated with EB virus. The EB virus belongs to the herpes group and there is some evidence to link another herpes virus (herpes simplex type II) with carcinoma of the cervix. Hepatitis B virus causes cirrhosis, and hepatoma develops in some of these cases. Because hepatomas also occur with non-viral cirrhosis, it is not clear whether it is the cirrhosis or the virus which causes the tumour. More recently, a retrovirus (RNA virus) has been found to be associated with T lymphocyte leukaemia in the Caribbean area and Japan.

Some non-infectious chronic inflammatory disorders result in neo-plasms. One example is hepatoma developing in alcoholic cirrhosis; another is carcinoma developing in a chronic peptic ulcer.

The induction of neoplasia

There have been major advances in our knowledge of the induction of neoplasia by the discovery of oncogenes. For many years it has been postulated that viral infections may bring into the cell genetic material which becomes incorporated into the host genome, inducing the cell to adopt the features of a tumour cell. This postulate was supported by the in-vitro demonstration of cultured normal cells being transformed into tumour cells and the viral gene being included in the host genetic information. Furthermore, when the viral gene was eliminated, the tumour cells reverted back to normal. It could be imagined that mutation of genes by chemical carcinogens or irradiation could also produce similar tumour transformation. DNA from tumour cells, transformed by the chemical carcinogen methylcholanthrene, was transferred to normal cells and these in turn underwent transformation to tumour cells. Subsequent isolation and analysis of DNA from transformed cells have revealed that the properties of transformation can be identified in discrete short segments of the DNA molecule, each carrying a single gene—an oncogene. This differs only slightly from the normal gene—a proto-oncogene—in some cases by the substitution of only one nucleotide, guanine in the proto-oncogene and thymine in the oncogene. As a result of this substitution, the oncogene directs the synthesis of an abnormal protein; evidence is now coming forward that one such substitution changes the protein reponsible for controlling cell growth to one stimulating the uncontrolled growth characteristic of tumour cells.

There are other mechanisms for the activation of proto-oncogenes into oncogenes; these include (a) transfer of the gene to another chromosome where it may be stimulated by the genes responsible for synthesis of immunoglobulins, and (b) production of excessive quantities of the proto-oncogene which results in it assuming the activity of an oncogene.

Several human tumours, including carcinoma of bladder, colon and lung and some connective tissue tumours, have now been shown to possess these oncogenes. It seems probable that some cells depend on the occurrence of more than one oncogene before developing into tumours and this may indicate that cancer develops by a number of separate steps. In support of this multistep development are many of the observations which gave rise to the *two-stage theory of carcinogenesis*. If chemical carcinogens such as dimethylbenzanthracene (DMBA) are applied to skin in sufficiently low doses, no tumours develop although they do so at higher dosage. If, following low-dose DMBA, the skin is irritated, for example by croton oil which does not in itself produce tumours, then neoplasms of the skin develop. It was postulated that the first low-dose carcinogen (DMBA) produces changes in the DNA of affected cells, referred to as *initiation* of the tumour. The second, non-specific, irritant converts this latent tumour into an actual neoplasm—a *promoter* of the tumour. The interval between these two events is known as the *latent period* and may last for several years. Although there is experimental evidence in animals to support this theory, direct evidence of its application to man is lacking. Many steps may be involved, but an alteration in DNA appears to be the necessary change which gives rise to a tumour.

Premalignant states

There are some disorders which give an individual a significantly greater risk than normal of developing an invasive tumour. It is helpful to think of them as two groups: (1) *clinical conditions* which are not in themselves neoplastic but in which tumours may develop, and (2) *lesions* which show identifiable histological abnormalities, the cells showing some of the features of malignant cells.

Precancerous clinical conditions

These include the hereditary states in which tumours develop, such as polyposis coli, retinoblastoma, xeroderma pigmentosa and also the hereditary immunodeficiency syndromes. Some hamartomas which are congenital (though not necessarily hereditary) can give rise to malignancy, e.g. chondrosarcoma may arise in multiple chondromatosis.

Acquired inflammatory, metabolic or toxic disorders may give rise to tumours. Ulcerative colitis, atrophic gastritis and cirrhosis can all be regarded as premalignant conditions even though tumours arise in only a minority of patients. Metabolic abnormalities such as hypersecretion of oestrogens are premalignant conditions in that they predispose to tumours, e.g. carcinoma of the endometrium or breast.

Premalignant lesions

These are identifiable pathological lesions showing histological abnormalities which have some of the features of malignancy. They often show some degree of hyperplasia and dysplasia and there is an increased cell turnover rate. Some of the epithelial lesions are so atypical that they have all the cytological characteristics of malignancy but still do not show invasion. These are often called carcinoma-in-situ. There are problems of definition here, and if one takes invasion as the touchstone of malignancy, then these lesions are premalignant only. Unfortunately, in some sites, such as the urinary bladder or the breast, the in-situ lesion has such a high risk of invasion developing that it is considered to be a carcinoma even when in-situ. Premalignant lesions also occur in non-epithelial tissues but they are more difficult to identify. The importance of finding a precancerous lesion is that if it is localized and is removed, then the development of an invasive tumour is prevented. A list of some examples of *pre-invasive lesions* is given below but they are further discussed in the section dealing with systemic pathology.

Cervix: dysplasia, carcinoma-in-situ (cervical intraepithelial neoplasia, CIN).
Endometrium: atypical hyperplasia.
Breast: epitheliosis, Paget's disease, intraduct and intralobular carcinoma.
Colon: adenomas and papillomas.
Urinary bladder: papilloma, pre-invasive papillary transitional cell carcinoma.
Skin: Bowen's disease, solar keratosis.

There are many clinical problems associated with premalignant states but one of the major difficulties is to assess the risk and interval before the development of invasive tumour. It is usually impossible to give a precise assessment of the chance of an invasive tumour developing in a particular case.

11

Pathological Effects of Ionizing Radiation

Ionizing radiations occur in two forms, particulate and electromagnetic.

Particulate radiations

These consist of α-particles, β-particles, neutrons and protons. α-particles are rapidly moving nuclei of helium atoms, which are emitted spontaneously by radioactive elements such as radium and thorium, or are produced by the bombardment of the elements helium and boron by neutrons. β-particles are rapidly moving electrons carrying either a negative or a positive (positrons) charge. They are emitted naturally from many radioactive elements, and can also be produced by passing high-tension currents through cathode ray tubes. Neutrons are electrically neutral particles which are present in all atoms other than hydrogen. They can be generated in atomic piles from such elements as uranium. Since these particles are electrically neutral, they can penetrate the electron cloud of an atom relatively easily and reach its nucleus. The alteration of the nucleus of certain elements which results from this penetration leads to the emission of active ionizing radiations. Protons are the positively charged nuclei of hydrogen atoms which can be accelerated to very high velocities in a cyclotron. α-particles and protons are relatively large and have little penetrating power. β-particles, being smaller, penetrate tissues to a greater, though still limited, distance, i.e. up to 2 mm of tissue. As already indicated, neutrons penetrate relatively easily.

Electromagnetic radiations

Energy in the form of electromagnetic radiation is produced when an orbiting extranuclear electron passes to a lower orbit. The wavelength of this radiation depends on the energy released, large changes in energy producing very short wavelength γ-rays, and smaller changes producing ultraviolet light. X-rays have a slightly longer wavelength than γ-rays. Laser radiation consists of narrow beams of monochromatic light.

The penetrating power of electromagnetic radiation depends on its wavelength. Hence, ultraviolet light has very little penetrating power, whereas γ-rays and x-rays are much more penetrating.

Ionizing radiations form part of the normal environment in small and usually harmless amounts. They come in part from the sun (solar or cosmic radiations), in part from traces of radioactive elements incorporated in the soil, and in manufactured articles such as bricks. They will also emanate from human bodies themselves—radioactive carbon, for example, exists in bones and its presence there has been used to estimate the age of those found archaeologically.

X-rays and γ-rays are the forms of ionizing radiation which are most used in clinical practice. β-particles, or electrons, are made use of in certain circumstances, i.e. when radioactive gold or the isotopes of phosphorus and iodine are employed. The radium and radon seeds sometimes inserted into tissues by surgeons are sources of x-rays and γ-rays. The amount of radiation used in x-ray diagnosis is much less than is used in radiotherapy.

The response of cells to ionizing radiations

When ionizing radiations pass through human tissue, they produce ionization in atoms and molecules which lie in their path. Electrons are ejected from some atoms and become attached to those nearby so that the electrical charges of the atoms becomes unbalanced. This may cause a disturbance in the molecular pattern, leading to a chemical change which in turn may bring about pathological biological effects. Many cytoplasmic enzymes, including SH enzymes and adenosine triphosphatase, are inactivated by irradiation. The ionizing power of any radioactive source is measured in terms of its effect on a standard quantity of air, and the unit of quantity is a roentgen (R). The absorbed dose of radiation energy in tissues is expressed in units of rads or grays (1 gray = 100 rads) and varies as the inverse square of the distance from the source.

Radiation affects cells most easily when they are undergoing mitosis. Its action has been shown to be more severe when local oxygen tension is high. As with other toxic agents, the harmful effects of ionizing radiations on tissue will depend on the degree of exposure. Very small quantities of radiations such as exist in the atmosphere have no harmful effect; even the much greater amounts used in x-ray diagnosis, whether in terms of photographic plates or of intravenous radioactive isotopes, such as ^{59}Fe and ^{51}Cr, can safely be given. The harmful effects of ionizing radiations are, however, cumulative, which is a good reason for reducing unnecessary exposure to a minimum.

The first biological effect of radiations on cells in mitosis which can be observed is one of temporary inhibition of mitosis followed, after an interval of time, by an increased rate of mitotic division, i.e. such a dose has a stimulating effect on growths. This effect of x-rays has been made use of clinically in the improvement of eczema of the skin. With increased quantities of radiation, cells completely lose their ability to undergo mitotic division, and with higher doses still, necrosis can be induced in the mature (non-dividing) cells. When the dose is such that mitotic activity is impaired but the cell remains viable, the visible histological effect is one of enlargement of the cell to a size greater than normal. The shape of the nucleus and the cell may also become abnormal because of partial derangement of essential cell functions. The visible harmful effects of radiations on cells may take time to appear; the higher the dose, the shorter the time. With doses used in radiotherapy it is not possible to say that an exposed cell, which looks healthy under the microscope, will not develop degenerative changes as a result of the x-rays until three months have elapsed since the completion of radiotherapy.

The tissues of the body vary very much in their sensitivity to a given quantum of radiation. The sensitivity bears a direct relationship to the natural mitotic activity of the component cells. The lymphoreticular tissue, the haemopoietic cells, germinal epithelium, squamous and gastrointestinal epithelium are the most radiosensitive; the central nervous system and all types of muscle are the most radioresistant, the remaining tissues occupying an intermediate place (radioresponsive).

As most tissues of the body consist of parenchyma and stroma, the total effect of radiation on the tissue is compounded of the direct action on the parenchyma and indirect action through the effect on the supporting connective tissue. A dose of radiation sufficient to inhibit mitotic activity in epithelium may stimulate fibrous tissue formation and the proliferation of the endothelial cells of the blood vessels. Both these effects will indirectly reduce the viability of the epithelial cells.

The response of malignant tissues to radiotherapy varies in the same way as that of the normal counterparts. However, as the rate of growth and hence the mitotic activity are usually above normal, malignant tumours are more sensitive than normal tissues to the effects of ionizing radiations, and this is the basic reason why this form of treatment is given for malignant disease. Another feature of malignant tumours is their tendency to be less well differentiated than the normal cells of the tissues from which they arise; in extreme cases the tumour cells can appear so undifferentiated that it is impossible under the microscope to determine their origin. This lack of differentiation, or anaplasia, is usually accompanied by increased radiosensitivity. However, this increased susceptibility is frequently more than counterbalanced by the increased tendency of the tumour to spread to other sites, and so beyond the range of radiotherapeutic control. Another point of difference in the response to radiotherapy of primary malignant tumours and recurrent or metastatic tumours is that, in the former, there is frequently a small number of malignant cells which are relatively resistant to the effects of the ionizing radiations. If these survive the first treatment, they multiply and lead to a recurrence of tumour which proves to be more radioresistant than the original one, and this increased resistance is progressive. It is for this reason that the treatment of many malignant tumours is more palliative than curative.

The results of overexposure to radiations

The complications of accidental overexposure to irradiation will depend on the quantum of incident radiations and the amount of tissues involved. The most frequent risk to overexposure occurs clinically during radiotherapy, because the margin between the amount of radiation required to kill malignant cells and the amount toxic to normal ones is small. During treatment, normal tissue is shielded as much as possible, but inevitably the skin lying over the part irradiated is subjected to the risk of overexposure. In early stages this may result in hyperaemia and soreness, as in any other type of burn, and a permanent dilatation of the superficial vessels may develop, which can be easily seen through the atrophic epidermis. Later, the combination of the direct and indirect effects of irradiation may lead to a radionecrotic ulcer. The floor of this consists of acellular fibrous tissue in which the capillary blood vessel lumens are practically obliterated by endothelial proliferation and the inflammatory response is less than might be expected. Malignant change in the irradiated skin, i.e. squamous cell carcinoma, is a further possible complication. This was not uncommon in the early days of the clinical use of x-rays, but the greater precautions taken against overexposure at the present time have considerably diminished its incidence.

Fibrosis is always liable to develop in the deeper tissues when these have had excessive amounts of radiation, and, in certain situations, such as the hilar regions of the lungs, may lead to considerable functional embarrassment, such as dyspnoea. Many people feel constitutionally ill after a major course of x-ray therapy, a consequence of the considerable tissue breakdown and disorder of normal functions which are the inevitable by-products of such treatment.

Exposure of the whole body to irradiation can take place in different ways, and everyone involved with the process is subjected to small amounts all the time (background irradiation). Those handling and conveying radioactive materials as part of their work are at risk of much greater exposure; patients who have irradiation over the whole body, as in the treatment of malignant lymph nodes, are at greater risk still; and the greatest risk of all comes to those exposed to nuclear warfare. The effects will depend on the amount and type of radiation received. In the case of atom bombs, the heat of the explosion will kill all close to it. Those farther away tend to die of a generalized illness, radiation sickness presumably resulting from the cessation of vital metabolic activities. Those farther away still may appear normal to begin with, but will eventually decline and die. This appears to be due to the effect on the radiosensitive reticuloendothelial system, leading on the one hand to inhibition of antibody production, and hence decreased resistance to infection, and on the other to an interference with normal blood formation resulting in aplastic anaemia. Platelet production is often affected earlier than red cell formation, so thrombocytopenic purpura may be the earliest manifestation of the aplastic anaemia.

It has been shown that in a proportion of those surviving exposure to an atomic explosion for some months there is an increased risk of developing leukaemia. This risk has also been shown to occur in those who are exposed more than normally to other sources of ionizing radiations. For instance, more radiologists have died from this disease than other physicians, and patients who have had a number of x-ray treatments to bone, as in ankylosing spondylitis, also have a higher incidence of the disease. Other malignant tumours that occur following irradiation include those in skin, thyroid, lung and breast. The gonads are also very susceptible to ionizing radiation, with the result that sterility has occurred in those exposed to the hazard. Cataracts develop in eyes exposed to high doses of irradiation. Experimentally it has been shown that the radiations can produce mutations as a result of alteration of genes, and abnormal chromosomes have been shown to occur in chronic myeloid leukaemia and other diseases. This points to the risks of congenital defects developing in the offspring of those people exposed to radiations in doses insufficient to produce sterility.

It is clear, because of the many hazards which arise as a result of exposure to ionizing radiations, that great care should be taken to minimize the dose received by those at risk. As the blood cells are affected early by ionizing radiations, regular blood counts were for a long time the means of keeping a check on overdose. It has come to be appreciated that these are not sensitive or exact enough measures and they have been replaced by the wearing of x-ray-sensitive photographic plates on coat lapels. This gives a quantitative measure of exposure, which is particularly important as it is known that the ill-effects of ionizing radiations are cumulative.

Part II

Systemic Pathology

12

Pathology of the Systems

The number of pages available for the description of the pathology of the systems, or special pathology, is limited, so the account in the following chapters cannot be comprehensive. Students must look to larger reference books for information about the more obscure diseases. The pathology of the illnesses most commonly seen in the wards and the autopsy room will be described here, and space will be given to those rarer entities only when a knowledge of their pathology is contributory to the understanding of general principles.

Table 4 (p. 96), compiled from the statistics of the Office of Population Censuses and Surveys for England and Wales for 1982, gives some indication of the relative frequency of fatal diseases in the various systems. These are crude figures of the causes of death, being based on information supplied on death certificates. Less than one-third of people come to autopsy when they die, so that most of the causes of death given are clinical diagnoses, which inevitably must vary considerably in accuracy. Even when autopsies have been performed, the reasons for the death of the patient are not always clarified. Notwithstanding these objections, some conclusions can be fairly drawn from large numbers, as in these circumstances the inaccuracies of individual diagnoses tend to be ironed out. Further, the statistics compiled from the various countries tend to be largely similar, except for factors due to differences of environment.

There are some observations to be made from Table 4. First, the overwhelming importance of diseases of the circulatory system as causes of death should be noted. Including cerebrovascular disease, they account for approximately half the total. This situation arises because a frequent cause of death in this group is what might be called degenerative cardiovascular disease, a feature linked with the process of ageing. The number of deaths due to this cause is increasing because, as a result of the considerable advances in clinical medicine, people are living longer now than their predecessors did. This is shown, for example, by the low position in the table occupied by death from infective diseases, a total of 2116, which is to be compared with 20 000 deaths from this cause 30 years ago. Much of this reduction is due to the improved treatment of tuberculosis, deaths from this cause falling from 16 000 in 1950 to 564 in 1982. These figures for infective diseases do not include those of respiratory origin

95

Table 4. Causes of death in England and Wales, 1982 (population 49 606 800).

	Male	Female	Total
All causes	290 166	291 695	581 861
Circulatory system	139 717	144 529	284 246
Ischaemic heart disease	88 716	65 889	154 605
Cerebrovascular disease	26 235	42 793	69 028
Hypertensive disease	2 276	2 884	5 160
Rheumatic heart disease	803	2 105	2 908
Neoplasms—all	70 026	62 422	132 448
1. Trachea, bronchus and lung	25 962	8 870	34 832
2. Large intestine (including anus)	7 596	8 412	16 008
3. Breast (female)	—	12 405	12 405
4. Stomach	5 978	4 233	10 211
5. Haemolymphatic	4 215	3 749	7 964
6. Pancreas	2 898	2 822	5 720
7. Prostate	5 291	—	5 291
8. Bladder	2 968	1 275	4 243
9. Ovary	—	3 577	3 577
10. Uterus (incl. cervix)	—	3 512	3 512
11. Kidney	1 242	749	1 991
12. Cervix uteri	—	1 932	1 932
13. Brain	1 149	893	2 042
Respiratory system (excluding neoplasms)	43 652	44 459	88 111
Pneumonia	22 611	33 918	56 529
Chronic bronchitis	11 153	4 443	15 596
Injury and poisoning	11 572	8 038	19 610
Road traffic accidents	3 684	1 557	5 241
Digestive system (excluding neoplasms)	7 053	9 403	16 456
Genitourinary (excluding neoplasms)	3 870	4 262	8 132
Nervous system	3 597	3 961	7 558
Mental disorder	1 225	2 532	3 757
Suicide	2 781	1 498	4 279
Metabolic, endocrine etc.	2 521	3 442	5 963
Diabetes mellitus	1 979	2 555	4 534
Infectious and parasitic diseases	1 138	978	2 116
Blood and blood-forming organs (excluding neoplasms)	629	959	1 588

such as influenza, bronchitis and pneumonia which do much to swell the figure for respiratory deaths and which have also steadily declined over recent years because of antibiotic therapy. The importance of neoplasms as a cause of death is to be noted, these diseases being responsible for 23% of the total, and coming second to those due to circulatory disorders.

Outstanding in importance amongst neoplasms are those arising in the bronchus and lung, particularly in men. In women the number of deaths due to neoplasms in the bronchus and lung is increasing: it is about three-quarters of the number of deaths from carcinoma of the breast, double the number from carcinoma of the stomach and four times as many as deaths due to carcinoma of the cervix. In 1982 there were 25 962 deaths in men alone due to carcinoma of the bronchus and lung. This compares with a total of 5241 deaths for all persons from road traffic accidents. One of the most impressive and alarming changes in the pattern of disease has been the increase in lung cancer in the past 20 years. In 1949, the death rate from lung cancer for males was approximately 350 per million male population. In 1969 it had risen to more than 1000 per million, and for the age group 65–74 it was nearly 6000 per million. For males the figures remained similar in 1982, but the female rate is increasing. Much of this increase can be attributed to cigarette smoking. Many of the deaths from chronic bronchitis and ischaemic heart disease are also associated with this habit. It will be found helpful to refer back to the common causes of death in dealing with the various systems to appreciate their relative importance in clinical practice.

13

The Circulatory System

Atheroma

This is an extremely common disorder affecting the arterial tree, being increasingly more liable to occur the older the patient, but not directly linked with the phenomenon of ageing, as it may be absent in some old people and very extensive in some who are relatively young. Not only is atheroma common, but it is pre-eminent among diseases liable to cause the death of the sufferer and, as is the case with many of the other lethal diseases, the precise pathogenesis is still unknown.

Macroscopic picture

The lesions of atheroma may be divided into three categories of fatty streak, plaque and complicated lesions. Superficial yellow fatty streaks are common in the intima of the aorta in children and young adults. There is an uncertain relation between these streaks and atheromatous plaques which give rise to clinical disease. Atheromatous plaques increase in severity and prevalence particularly after the age of 35 years in men and 55 years in women. With more severe disease, complications develop with calcification or haemorrhage in the plaque, surface thrombosis and ulceration.

The atheromatous plaque is a focal swelling involving the intima of the aorta and its main branches, the coronary arteries and the cerebral arteries. The abdominal aorta immediately above the bifurcation is the part most liable to be involved, though plaques surrounding the orifices of the small branches leading off it are often early features. The uncomplicated plaque is yellow or cream coloured, firm with a smooth endothelial surface. When calcified it forms a hard plaque or it may appear brown if there has been haemorrhage into it or thrombosis on its surface; more severe lesions may ulcerate. When not calcified the fatty material has the consistency of paste. Cross-sections of coronary arteries show that the plaques form a crescent resulting in a narrowed and eccentric lumen. The media of large arteries is not directly affected, but it may become thin beneath the thickened intimal plaques due to impairment of oxygen diffusing from the lumen. This leads to fibrous replacement of the muscle with destruction of elastic tissue which may result in an aneurysm, a phenomenon most frequently seen at the distal end of the aorta.

Microscopic picture

The superficial fatty streaks show accumulation of fat droplets in smooth muscle cells and foamy macrophages in the subendothelial connective tissue. The established plaque shows eccentric proliferation of modified smooth muscle cells (myofibroblasts) which have infiltrated into the intima from the media. These cells are associated with deposition of collagen, elastic fibres and proteoglycans in the intima. Lipid continues to accumulate deep in the intima and between intimal collagen fibres. Gradually the fatty material becomes amorphous, and there is cellular necrosis. Capillaries grow into the plaque, mainly from the media, but also from the intima. The lipid deposited in the plaque is largely low-density lipoprotein, rich in cholesterol, which appears in histological sections as sharp-pointed clefts where the crystals have dissolved out in the processing of the tissue.

In the same area there is frequently evidence of extravasation of blood in the form of fibrin and free red cells or, where the latter have been broken down, in the form of brown granules of haemosiderin within histiocytes. Where fat and haemorrhage are present, calcification is common. Ulceration of the intimal surface causes thrombosis and subsequent organization. The underlying media is thinner due to partial fibrous replacement of the elastica and muscle. Aneurysm formation is associated with the formation on the luminal aspect of laminated organizing thrombus. In the adventitia there is commonly infiltration by chronic inflammatory cells around the vasa vasorum. This is seen particularly if the aneurysm is adherent to surrounding structures.

Complications

In addition to the formation of an aneurysm, the complications of atheroma mainly arise from the reduction of blood supply to the part concerned. This blood supply may become gradually reduced because the increasing amount of atheromatous change slowly narrows the lumen of the artery, or it may become suddenly shut off because of a subintimal haematoma in an atheromatous plaque or through the formation of an obliterative thrombus.

An embolus may form from a mural thrombus overlying a plaque, or the paste-like contents of a plaque may embolize if the surface ulcerates. The embolus may impact farther down the arterial tree. A gradual reduction of blood supply leads to replacement fibrosis in the part supplied, a sudden cut-off to infarction. These complications make their clinical impact mainly in three situations: (a) the heart, (b) the brain, and (c) the legs.

The heart: myocardial fibrosis and infarction

Atheroma is common in the coronary arteries, and more so in the left artery than in the right, the area of greatest severity being situated within

2–3 cm of the ostium of the left coronary artery and in the anterior descending branch; the left circumflex branch is least commonly involved.

Progressive narrowing of the arteries leads to the clinical syndrome of angina pectoris. This form of pain arises because the cardiac muscle is ischaemic, as a result of which it will show replacement fibrosis. Grey streaks may therefore be visible in the affected myocardium, and microscopically strands of fibrous tissue will be seen to run between the atrophic myocardial fibres. Occlusive thrombosis is a relatively common event in the coronary arteries, and is a frequent cause of death. The effect on the heart will depend on the site of the occlusion, and the extent of atheroma in the coronary artery system. Healthy coronary arteries act more or less as end-arteries, but the more narrowed they become as a result of atheroma, the more their terminal branches tend to anastomose with each other. In most instances, when occlusive thrombosis occurs, there is evidence of widespread atheroma throughout the coronary arteries. Coronary artery occlusion (or coronary thrombosis) leads to myocardial infarction which has a regional distribution according to the area supplied by the affected coronary artery. The most common site is the anterior aspect of the left ventricle and the anterior two-thirds of the interventricular septum, particularly in the region of the apex since this is the area supplied by the anterior descending branch of the left coronary artery. Infarcts rarely affect the right ventricle unless this has undergone hypertrophy. Poor perfusion of the coronary arteries, such as in hypotension, triple artery disease and after coronary bypass operations, may result in widespread infarction of the subendocardial zone of the left ventricular myocardium — a laminar infarct. The infarction may lead to immediate cardiac failure, and, indeed, this is a common cause of sudden death. Under these circumstances no change will be visible in the myocardium. If the patient survives the initial period after infarction and dies a little later, the affected myocardium will show changes, the picture depending on the time interval between thrombosis and the death of the patient. After 6–12 hours, loss of enzyme activity in the damaged myocardium may be demonstrated. Two to three days later the infarcted myocardium becomes yellowish brown, surrounded by a haemorrhagic zone. After two to three weeks, white fibrous tissue gradually replaces the dead muscle.

A healed infarct will consist of a fibrous scar. If the infarct reaches the pericardium, this will become inflamed and covered with a fibrinous exudate (fibrinous pericarditis), leading eventually to fibrous adhesions between the visceral and parietal pericardium. On the endocardial surface, damage to the endocardium and lack of movement of the dead muscle allow platelet adhesion and the formation of a mural thrombus in the recesses of the muscular trabeculae.

There are complications of myocardial infarction other than death from acute cardiac failure. The infarction may be superimposed on an already fibrotic myocardium, so that chronic cardiac failure may ensue. The endocardial mural thrombi may break off into the circulation, and the resulting emboli may lead to the formation of infarcts in other organs, of which the most important clinically is the brain. The infarcted myocardium is softened in the earlier stages and may rupture, leading to the formation of a haemopericardium with resultant death from cardiac tamponade. Under these circumstances the chambers of the heart are unable to fill during diastole. Alternatively the rupture may involve the interventricular septum, causing a ventricular septal defect, or it may result in rupture of a papillary muscle and sudden mitral incompetence. The fibrous scar of a healed infarct may make the myocardial wall so thin that aneurysmal dilatation occurs with subsequent risk of rupture. This is most likely to take place at the apex where the myocardium is normally thinner than elsewhere. Other complications of myocardial ischaemia include cardiac arrhythmias. Atrial fibrillation may result in the formation of thrombi in the atrial appendage with the risk of emboli from this site. An infarct may involve the conducting system, resulting in heart block.

The brain: cerebral thrombosis and embolism

Cerebral infarction is a relatively common lesion in adults and is usually due to atheroma. It may follow occlusion of a branch of one of the cerebral arteries, most commonly the middle cerebral. However, it may also follow occlusion of the internal carotid artery just beyond its origin from the common carotid artery in the neck. Many cerebral infarcts follow embolism into a cerebral artery by a fragment of thrombus or atheromatous debris from one of these larger, more proximal arteries.

The legs: intermittent claudication and infarction

The gradual narrowing of the main arteries in the legs as a result of atheroma leads to the symptoms of intermittent claudication, or muscular pain in the calves on exercise. No pathological changes can usually be identified in the limb except for the severe atheroma. Occlusion of a proximal segment of the arterial supply to the legs may not produce any further symptoms because blood passes through collateral arteries. Occlusion of one of the more distal branches, however, may result in infarction of the part of the foot supplied.

Aneurysm formation

This relatively uncommon but important complication of atheroma has already been mentioned (see above). It occurs most frequently at the distal end of the aorta below the renal arteries, and may reach the size of a hen's egg or larger. The aneurysm may either leak blood slowly or may rupture producing more acute abdominal symptoms.

Aetiology

Though the disease is extremely common, there is still doubt about the factors associated with its development. No one factor can be held responsible and it seems probable that there is a cumulative effect of several predisposing factors.

Blood lipids

The lipids which accumulate in atheromatous plaques are thought to originate in the blood. Lipids are normally carried in the blood as complexes with protein in the form of lipoproteins. These may be classified into chylomicrons of large size, rich in triglycerides, and three subclasses divided according to their density and electrophoretic mobility—high-density lipoproteins (HDL or α-lipoproteins), low-density lipoproteins (LDL or β-lipoproteins), and very low-density lipoproteins (VLDL or pre-β-lipoproteins). It is the last two which are associated with the development of atheroma, whereas there is a mechanism for clearing HDL from the vessel wall. The ratio of LDL to HDL is important in the development of atheroma. This ratio is increased by a diet rich in animal (saturated) fats and refined carbohydrates and it is lowered by a diet containing largely polyunsaturated vegetable and fish fats. The high incidence of atheroma in the Western Hemisphere may partly be accounted for by the high concentration of animal fat and sugar in the diet. The LDL to HDL ratio is also increased in diabetes mellitus, myxoedema and in some forms of familial hyperlipoproteinaemias. Recent evidence has indicated that it is possible to reduce the risk of developing coronary heart disease in patients with a high blood cholesterol level by giving a diet with a high polyunsaturated : saturated fat ratio together with oral cholestyramine to prevent reabsorption of bile salts. This regime lowers the plasma LDL levels and produces a small rise in protective HDL.

Age

The disease increases in frequency with age, but the correlation is not absolute, for it may be minimal in old age and severe in the young.

Sex

Men are more frequently affected than women, although the incidence increases rapidly in women after the menopause.

Hypertension

Atheroma is more frequent in association with hypertension and this applies particularly in the pulmonary circulation. However, atheroma may be severe in normotensive individuals or absent in those with severe hypertension, particularly in black Africans, in whom dietary factors may be protective.

Mechanical stress

Atheromatous plaques tend to be localized and most severe at the bifurcation of large arteries or at the ostia of small branches where turbulence is greatest.

Cigarette smoking

There is a higher incidence of ischaemic heart disease in cigarette smokers but the relation to atheroma is complex. There is evidence to suggest that smoking increases platelet adhesiveness and this may be the basis for increased coronary artery thrombosis.

Pathogenesis

There are two principal theories of the development of atheroma. The *imbibition or filtration theory* relates atheroma to blood lipid, particularly to the level of β-lipoprotein. This theory postulates that relatively insoluble lipid passes into the vessel wall from the lumen. Because of the absence of blood and lymph capillaries from the intima, the lipid accumulates in the deep intima. However, this theory requires additional factors to explain the localization of atheromatous lesions within vessels. It is postulated that local mechanical factors (such as turbulence of blood) cause the localization of the lesions and this can be demonstrated experimentally. Once fat is deposited in the intima it induces the fibrous reaction forming part of the atheromatous plaque.

The *incrustation or thrombogenic theory* suggests that atheroma is due to thrombi being deposited on the vessel wall. Initially these consist of platelets and fibrin. The foam cells of the early lesion represent histiocytes which have phagocytosed platelets rich in lipoprotein. When mural thrombi have formed they become covered by endothelium, the blood breaks down to give the cholesterol and blood pigment, while organization of the thrombus gives rise to the fibrous tissue. This theory explains the irregular distribution of atheroma in the body and the eccentric lesion in the vessel. It is probable that both these theories are involved in the production of the established lesion.

A third theory in the development of atheroma is the *monoclonal proliferation of myofibroblasts*. Some people, particularly American black females, are heterozygous for the X-linked genes responsible for the formation of the isoenzymes of glucose-6-phosphate dehydrogenase. As a result they produce two isoenzymes, A and B. Examination of the atheromatous plaques from these patients reveals that some myofibroblasts are exclusively A and in other plaques they are B, suggesting that they have arisen by the monoclonal proliferation of myofibroblasts of one or other type. This raises the possibility of neoplastic proliferation of the myofibroblasts in these plaques, although there are other explanations including selective proliferation of one type with suppression or destruction of the other.

The incidence of atheroma does not appear to have altered much in the past 50 years, but the incidence of coronary thrombosis has greatly increased. This suggests that other factors, increasing the tendency to thrombosis, may be important in the genesis of coronary occlusion. In this connection it is noteworthy that some lipids are augmentors of blood coagulation, and that platelets have been shown to be more sticky than normal in this disease.

Hypertension

Definition

Hypertension means a raised blood pressure. There is still no general agreement for a blood pressure figure which represents the upper limit of normal, partly because it may fluctuate under emotional and other stresses, partly because it increases with age, and partly because its measurement is commonly not wholly objective. The diastolic pressure reading is considered to be more important than the systolic, and a persistent level of over 100 mmHg should be regarded with suspicion.

Aetiology

Hypertension most commonly exists without any coexistent disease— *essential hypertension*; where an underlying cause is recognized, the hypertension is said to be *secondary*. The most significant aetiological factor is renal disease and for this the term *renal hypertension* is used. The commoner renal diseases involved are proliferative glomerulonephritis, pyelonephritis, and scarring due to analgesic abuse. Experimentally hypertension may be produced by creating renal ischaemia by clamping a renal artery. The counterpart in human disease, renal artery stenosis, is rare. Other renal diseases which give rise to hypertension include polycystic kidneys, and amyloidosis. There are many *endocrine* causes of hypertension. A tumour of the adrenal medulla (phaeochromocytoma) which is capable of secreting noradrenaline and adrenaline excessively may at first give rise to intermittent hypertension, followed by sustained hypertension. Although uncommon, this is an important diagnosis because surgery can effect a cure if undertaken before irreversible renal damage has been caused by the hypertension. Tumours of the adrenal cortex, leading either to excess production of glucocorticoids and Cushing's syndrome, or to the excessive production of aldosterone and Conn's syndrome, may also cause hypertension. Sometimes the cause is due to hyperplasia of the adrenal cortex rather than neoplasm.

Dietary salt intake is also considered to be an important aetiological factor in the production of hypertension. Another important cause is *toxaemia of pregnancy*, but the precise mechanism is uncertain. Finally, *congenital malformations* such as coarctation of the aorta may give rise to hypertension proximal to the obstruction.

In most of these cases the disease persists for several years and in many instances it is silent until an advanced stage. It is referred to as *benign hypertension* but this is a misnomer as it frequently is the cause of death. *Malignant or accelerated hypertension* is diagnosed if a patient suffers from a rapidly increasing blood pressure, which is associated with the presence of papilloedema, retinal haemorrhages and exudate, and renal failure.

Pathology

The blood pressure is the product of cardiac output and peripheral resistance. In hypertension from all causes, the important factor is increased peripheral resistance. In the early stages of the disease, no structural changes can be identified, so that the diagnosis remains clinical. This finding also indicates that the first change is a functional narrowing of the smaller blood vessels. When structural changes appear, the first elements to become altered (as might be expected) are the distal components of the arterial tree, the arterioles. The walls of these vessels become thickened and the lumens narrowed. The thickening is partly due to hypertrophy of muscle, and partly to deposition of plasma proteins and lipids deep to the endothelium. Characteristically a glassy eosinophilic change supervenes—*hyaline arteriolosclerosis*. This change can take place throughout the body, but, perhaps significantly, it only has a high correlation with the development of hypertension when observed in the kidney. By contrast, similar changes in the arterioles of the Malpighian corpuscles of the spleen are common, and are of no hypertensive significance. The development in other viscera is of intermediate significance.

The primary arteriolar sclerosis in the *kidney* causes two further changes. First, because of the increased peripheral resistance, the arteries undergo hypertrophy in an attempt to compensate for it. The thickening of the artery walls can be appreciated macroscopically, because the cut surfaces tend to be much more prominent than normal. Microscopically, three elements of the artery contribute to its increase of size. The muscle coat hypertrophies, there is a concentric new formation of fibrous tissue in the intima, and the internal elastic lamina reduplicates, or splits into two or more layers. Secondly, because of the narrowed arteriolar lumens, the blood supply becomes reduced to the tissues distally. An arteriole supplies a small number of nephrons, and these will undergo ischaemic collapse and sclerosis. Since the tubules are supplied via the glomerular efferent arterioles, these also became ischaemic and atrophied as the glomeruli are sclerosed, leaving a fibrous scar. Not all arterioles are affected equally, so that small foci of fibrous tissue are interspersed between normal surviving nephrons, which may in fact show compensatory hyperplasia. The result of these changes is the production of the characteristic finely granular capsular surface of the kidney, slight loss of detail in the cut surface, and moderate reduction in the overall size of this organ. The kidney of essential hypertension is thus one of the causes of contracted granular kidney. The arcuate and larger arteries will be more prominent than normal when the cut surface of the kidney is examined.

In order to maintain an adequate blood flow in the face of increasing peripheral resistance, the left ventricle of *the heart* eventually undergoes hypertrophy, which may in time become very striking (cor bovinum). The left ventricular cavity usually remains relatively small unless cardiac failure supervenes.

Malignant hypertension can exist without demonstrable arterial lesions. There are two changes which are characteristic of this state. First, the renal arterioles and intraglomerular capillaries may show fibrinoid change. This is similar histologically to hyaline arteriolosclerosis but tends to be a deeper pink and is, in fact, due to deposition of fibrin and fibrinogen, often mixed with fragmented red blood cells deep to the endothelium. It is believed to be due to intravascular coagulation as a result of the hypertension possibly damaging endothelial cells. Endothelium subsequently overgrows the fibrin thrombus and so incorporates it into the vessel wall. Similar changes may be seen in other conditions associated with intravascular coagulation. The second vascular lesion of malignant hypertension is a very loose lamellated ('onion-skin') mucoid thickening of the arterial wall. In very small vessels, such as in the retina, there may be necrosis of muscle cells. Where the arteriolar walls are necrotic, small haemorrhages are liable to develop, and when the blood supply to the distal tissues is reduced rather rapidly, small infarcts may arise.

Complications

The majority of people with essential hypertension eventually suffer from, and die of, *heart failure*. A common episode is acute left ventricular failure, the development of a sudden crisis of dyspnoea because the failure precipitates pulmonary oedema. Frequently, however, the failure is more gradual, the strain being taken up by both ventricles so that ultimately congestive cardiac failure develops. *Apoplexy or cerebral haemorrhage* is the next most common complication of essential hypertension. This is most frequently seen in the region of the internal capsule and may be of considerable extent. Such a haemorrhage may be accompanied by other small haemorrhages elsewhere in the brain and are related to the formation and rupture of intracerebral microaneurysms as a result of hypertension.

Chronic renal failure is less common than the other two complications in essential hypertension, but, in malignant hypertension, death is most frequently by way of uraemia. In addition to the effects of hypertension, there is often severe atheroma which further complicates the cardiac, cerebral and renal disease.

Mechanism

Much of the experimental work on renal hypertension indicates that renal ischaemia plays an important role. Clamping of one renal artery results in hypertension, but if the clamp is removed before vascular changes have developed in the opposite kidney, the hypertension resolves. However, if release of the clamp is delayed, the hypertension is rreversible. It has been shown that an inactive pressor substance, renin, is produced by the juxtaglomerular cells of the afferent arterioles as they enter glomerular tufts in the renal cortex. Renin acts on a circulating globulin, angiotensinogen, to produce angiotensin I. This is further broken down in the lungs to angiotensin II which has a direct effect on arterioles causing vasoconstriction and leading to hypertension. It also stimulates the production of aldosterone by the adrenal cortex and this aldosterone leads to sodium and water retention contributing to the hypertension. However, in most cases of hypertension renin levels are not raised. In Conn's syndrome (adrenal cortical adenoma producing aldosterone) renin levels are low.

Other factors may also play an important part, particularly neurogenic factors. Elevation of the blood pressure can be shown to follow emotional stimulation. Sympathectomy is effective in reducing the blood pressure in a number of patients. It may be that in essential hypertension, emotional stimulation causes the initial hypertension, and the resulting arterial disease causes renal damage which perpetuates the hypertension.

Rheumatic heart disease

Rheumatic heart disease is an illness which appears to be less common in developed countries than it used to be, although it is still common in Third World countries. The *acute attack* (acute rheumatism) is a delayed inflammatory reaction following an infection by *Streptococcus pyogenes* (see p. 14). It affects the heart, the joints and the nervous system. In the heart all layers are involved. The endocardium is the seat of a chronic inflammatory reaction, mainly in the region of the valves, though the posterior wall of the left atrium is often also implicated (McCallum's patch). The naked-eye evidence of inflammation is the presence of small wart-like vegetations measuring about 1 mm in diameter and composed largely of platelet clumps and fibrin. On the valves, these lie along the line of closure. The valves on the left side of the heart are much more commonly affected than those on the right, and the mitral valve more frequently than the aortic. More than one valve can be affected in an individual patient. No naked-eye change can be identified in the myocardium, though it is here that the characteristic Aschoff nodes occur. These are found in the loose perivascular connective tissue of the myocardium and consist of fibrinoid necrosis surrounded by histiocytic mesenchymal cells (Anitschkow myocytes), lymphocytes and giant cells. As the lesion heals it leaves a fibrous scar. Fibrinous pericarditis may develop and results in an adherent pericardium. Joints are commonly involved but rarely give permanent disability. There are focal areas of mucoid or fibrinoid change in the synovium, and sometimes lesions resembling Aschoff nodes. In the subcutaneous tissues, especially around joints, rheumatic nodules may form. These are similar to nodules found in rheumatoid arthritis and consist of fibrinoid necrosis surrounded by palisaded histiocytes and lymphocytes. The lungs may show interstitial pneumonitis and there may be lymphocytic perivascular cuffing of vessels in the brain associated with chorea. Acute rheumatism of the heart may heal, but this recovery carries with it an increased risk of subsequent attacks compared with normal people. Some cases will die of acute cardiac failure; on the other hand, acute rheumatic fever may develop over the years into chronic rheumatic heart disease. The latter may also appear unexpectedly in an individual who cannot recollect having had rheumatic fever.

Chronic rheumatic heart disease is dominated by a progressive sclerosis of valvular endocardium. The mitral valve is most frequently affected. The valve cusps thicken and fuse, and the chordae tendineae shorten, thicken, become paler and sometimes matted. Mitral stenosis thus develops with a rigid orifice, and there may be in addition calcification of the valve leaflets. Such stenotic valves are inevitably also incompetent, but the disease occasionally leads to such rigidity of the valve leaflets that incompetence becomes the dominant feature.

The aortic valve is also frequently affected in chronic rheumatic heart disease. The aortic valve cusps adhere at their contiguous edges, and when the sclerotic cusps shrink towards their points of attachment, incompetence results. The valve becomes stenosed rather than incompetent when the tendency of the cusps to adhere dominates over their tendency to retract. Superadded calcification sometimes complicates the stenosis.

Lesions are much less common in the valves of the right side of the heart. The tricuspid valve may show functional incompetence when severe mitral stenosis leads to pulmonary congestion followed by pulmonary hypertension and right ventricular failure.

The diseased valves throw a strain on the heart and changes develop, particularly in the pulmonary circulation. The obstruction to flow through the mitral valve causes dilatation of the left atrium and hypertrophy of the atrial muscle. When atrial fibrillation intervenes, thrombus is very liable to form in the atrial appendage and this may break off to form an embolus in the systemic circulation. Back pressure on the pulmonary circulation causes congestion of the lungs and the escape of red blood cells in the alveoli. The haemoglobin is broken down to haemosiderin where it may be seen in macrophages—'heart-failure cells'. The chronic congestion stimulates fibrous proliferation in the alveolar walls, and this thickening, together with the haemosiderin pigmentation, gives rise to the macroscopic appearance of 'brown induration' of the lungs. When pulmonary hypertension is severe, atheroma develops in the pulmonary artery. Disease of the aortic valve results in dilatation and hypertrophy of the left ventricle, and when this fails pulmonary oedema develops. Another important complication of chronic rheumatic heart disease is bacterial endocarditis.

Endocarditis

In the past, infective endocarditis was subdivided into subacute bacterial endocarditis and acute bacterial endocarditis. The former usually ran a protracted course and was due to infection with organisms of low virulence, usually in a heart previously damaged by, for example, congenital malformation or rheumatic valvular disease. Acute bacterial endocarditis was a fulminating illness, fatal after a short period of illness, and due to pyogenic organisms of high virulence which caused rapid destruction of heart valves. The course of these illnesses has been modified by antibiotic therapy, by drug therapy which modifies the immune response, by cardiac surgery and, in drug addicts, by introducing other micro-organisms during intravenous injections. Patterns of infective endocarditis intermediate between the two classical forms are now seen and the range of micro-organisms has increased to include fungi (*Candida* and *Aspergillus*), rickettsiae (*Coxiella burnetii*) and chlamydiae (*C. psittaci*). Nevertheless, in spite of these modifications, it is still of value to use the terms subacute and acute bacterial endocarditis.

Acute bacterial endocarditis, which is rare, is a terminal event in a severe acute septicaemic infection, originating elsewhere in the body and caused usually by *Staphylococcus aureus*, and less commonly by *Strep. pneumoniae*, β-haemolytic streptococci or gonococci. The infection may affect either healthy or previously diseased valves. The vegetations are larger and more crumbly than in acute rheumatism, tending to ulcerate the affected cusps and chordae tendineae and to erode into the underlying myocardium. They consist of platelets and fibrin but include clumps of bacteria, and inflammatory cells. The friable vegetations are very liable to break off to form emboli which lead to the formation of infected infarcts which tend to suppurate. Untreated, the patients do not survive long, either because of the septicaemia or the destructive endocarditis.

Subacute bacterial endocarditis is different from the acute form in the pathogenicity of the infecting organisms. The disease has an insidious onset and, when untreated, a protracted course. The patient may present as a pyrexia of unknown origin (PUO) which may be accompanied by symptoms due to embolic phenomena. The disease is due to infection with *Streptococcus viridans*, a relatively avirulent organism, in the majority of cases. This gets into the bloodstream transiently in normal people from the region of the teeth during mastication, but is more liable to do so if dental caries is present. In affected patients, the organisms settle in the valves because they are diseased, the two principal abnormalities being chronic rheumatic heart disease and, in the case of the aorta, congenitally bicuspid valves. The orifice of a patent ductus arteriosus or the endocardium overlying the myocardium adjacent to a diseased valve or congenital malformation may also be infected. Because of the decreased incidence of chronic rheumatic heart disease and of improved dental hygiene, the disease is not so common as it used to be. Its previous gloomy prognosis has been ameliorated by the advent of antibiotic therapy. The vegetations are large and crumbly like the acute ones, but are often more extensive because of the longer course of the disease. The microscopic structure of the vegetations is similar to that in the acute form, except that they show the features of organization at the point of attachment to the valve. Extension to the left atrial endocardium may occur as in rheumatic heart disease. Erosion and ulceration of the valve cusps are less common complications than in acute bacterial endocarditis, embolization tending to dominate the scene. The brain, spleen, kidney and skin are common sites for the emboli, which, in contrast to those of the acute disease, do not suppurate. This is because the organism is less virulent, and also antibodies have been able to develop to high titre. In addition to emboli which occlude medium-sized arteries, some patients develop proliferative glomerulonephritis due to the deposition of immune complexes of antigen and antibody in the glomerular capillary wall.

Other manifestations of the disease include splenomegaly, splinter haemorrhages beneath the nails, tender nodules in the pulp of fingers and toes (Osler's nodes), and finger clubbing.

Other forms of endocarditis

Verrucous endocarditis or *Libman–Sacks endocarditis* is due to systemic lupus erythematosus. Small vegetations occur on the mitral and tricuspid valves and, less frequently, on the semilunar valves. The vegetations may occur anywhere on the cusps, but they differ from those of rheumatic fever in that they may extend on to the undersurface of the cusp. The valves show mucoid change and foci of fibrinoid necrosis, later leading to fibroblastic proliferation.

Non-bacterial, thrombotic endocarditis is found in patients dying after protracted debilitating diseases such as advanced malignancy. The vegetations are found particularly on the mitral and aortic valves and consist largely of fibrin and platelets. They are thought to occur as an agonal event.

Carcinoid syndrome due to excessive secretion of 5-hydroxytryptamine, usually by metastatic carcinoid tumour arising in the ileum, gives rise to widespread fibrous thickening of the endocardium in the right side of the heart. This fibrosis results in pulmonary stenosis.

Floppy mitral valve syndrome is associated with mucoid degeneration of the valve cusps, the posterior being affected more than the anterior. During ventricular systole, the valve cusp balloons back into the left atrium and may lead to mitral incompetence. There is an association with Marfan's syndrome.

Other lesions of the heart

Myocarditis

Sudden death may occasionally be due to myocarditis. It may be possible to identify the infecting organisms and these include: (1) pyogenic bacteria in cases of septicaemia, (2) bacteria causing diphtheria, where the damage is due to the exotoxin of the bacteria producing fatty degeneration of the cardiac muscle, (3) viruses, especially Coxsackie B and those causing poliomyelitis, measles and mumps, and (4) parasites such as *Toxoplasma* and *Trypanosoma* (the latter causing Chagas' disease). Other forms of myocarditis, for example sarcoidosis, may not be associated with an identifiable infective agent.

Cardiomyopathy

This term is used to describe myocardial disease which is not attributed to ischaemia, hypertension, acquired valvular disease, congenital heart disease or myocarditis. Various classifications are available, but a simple one is as follows.

1. Hypertrophic obstructive cardiomyopathy (HOCM).
2. Congestive cardiomyopathy.
3. Obliterative cardiomyopathy.
4. Restrictive cardiomyopathy.

Hypertrophic obstructive cardiomyopathy is a cause of sudden death in young people. There is asymmetrical hypertrophy of the left ventricle, often affecting the septum to give obstruction to the left ventricular outflow. The function of the heart is also affected by increased rigidity of the left ventricular myocardium. *Congestive cardiomyopathy* results in congestive cardiac failure, often associated with mural thrombus in the ventricle. Both of these conditions may show a familial incidence. Congestive cardiomyopathy is also associated with chronic alcoholism, beri-beri and haemochromatosis.

Two conditions are associated with *obliterative cardiomyopathy*. Endomyocardial fibrosis affects both right and left sides of the heart. Many of the features resemble those of organized thrombus resulting in obliteration of the ventricular lumen. This is a disease seen in African children but has some features in common with Loeffler's endocarditis which is associated with pronounced blood eosinophilia and may be related to parasitic infestation. The second condition giving obliterative cardiomyopathy is endocardial fibroelastosis which usually presents in early infancy with widespread thickening of the endocardium. It has been suggested that this may be due to viral infection or fetal anoxia.

Restrictive cardiomyopathy is seen in amyloid infiltration which occurs in primary amyloidosis and in amyloidosis associated with multiple myeloma.

Pericarditis

The fibrinous pericarditis of acute rheumatism and myocardial infarction have already been mentioned. Bacterial pericarditis may complicate acute inflammatory conditions of the lungs. Pericarditis is also a terminal complication of uraemia. It is a feature of malignant tumour infiltration, usually from the lung. Chronic pericarditis is a feature of tuberculosis and can also arise without known aetiology (chronic constrictive pericarditis).

Macroscopically, the changes of acute or chronic inflammation will be seen, with an exudate forming in the cavity, being serofibrinous or fibrinopurulent in the acute cases, caseous or fibrinous in tuberculosis, and haemorrhagic in malignant cases. Small pericardial effusions are common events in the post-mortem room. They are transudates, usually due to the causes of generalized oedema, e.g. cardiac failure.

Tumours

Primary tumours of the heart are very rare. 'Rhabdomyomas' of the cardiac muscle are hamartomas sometimes found in patients with tuberose sclerosis. Atrial myxomas arise in the vicinity of the interatrial septum, more commonly on the left. They are usually polypoid tumours and may block the mitral orifice when the patient is erect. Secondary tumours especially those arising in the lung, commonly infiltrate the pericardium and myocardium.

Congenital heart disease

This is an important cause of perinatal mortality, but minor grades are compatible with adult life. Only the more common disorders are mentioned. *Fallot's tetralogy* consists of a subvalvular pulmonary stenosis with a ventricular septal defect, an overriding aorta and right ventricular hypertrophy. As deoxygenated blood from the right ventricle enters the aorta, there is cyanosis of varying degree. *Eisenmenger's complex* is similar, without pulmonary stenosis. *Patent foramen ovale*, as a valvular defect, is a common finding at post-mortem. When there are large *atrial or ventricular septal defects* the shunt of blood is usually from left to right. In *patent ductus arteriosus* the ductus is normally obliterated by eight weeks of extra-uterine life, but when it remains patent it allows a shunt of blood from the aorta to the pulmonary artery. *Coarctation of the aorta* is a constriction most commonly between the origin of the left subclavian artery and the ductus arteriosus, but occasionally occurring in other situations. It may be associated with a bicuspid aortic valve. The complications of congenital heart disease include cardiac failure, pulmonary hypertension, cyanosis, hypertrophic pulmonary osteoarthropathy and subacute bacterial endocarditis.

Syphilitic aortitis

This has become much less common in recent years, largely because of the response of syphilis to therapy with penicillin. The first part of the aorta above the level of the diaphragm is most commonly affected; the aorta appears dilated and thin. The intima is usually the seat of extensive atheroma, but between the fibrous plaques it is characteristically wrinkled. Histologically there is intense cuffing of the vasa vasorum of the aorta by chronic inflammatory cells, particularly plasma cells. The lumina of these small vessels tend to be obliterated by reactive thickening of the walls, so that the blood supply, and hence the nutrition of the aortic media, is impaired. As a consequence, there is degeneration of the elastic and muscle fibres with replacement of the media by vascular scar tissue.

Syphilitic aortitis which proceeds only to minor dilatation of the vessel does not lead to the development of symptoms. These will arise only if the aortic valve ring is involved or if an aneurysm develops in the aorta. The valve ring is, in fact, commonly affected, and its dilatation leads to incompetence of the valve. This change can be inferred to have occurred if the commissures between the valve leaflets are seen to be wider than normal. The leaflets themselves may become somewhat fibrotic. The aortic incompetence means that some of the blood expelled into the aorta during systole regurgitates into the left ventricle during diastole at a time when it is receiving blood from the lungs by way of the left atrium. The left ventricle enlarges, partly because it becomes more dilated to accommodate the increased amount of blood during diastole, and partly because it hypertrophies in order to expel the greater load in systole. Left ventricular failure is thus a common end-result in this disease. If the destruction of the elastic coat of the aorta by syphilis is sufficiently severe at any point, a saccular aneurysm develops. The aneurysm, as it grows, is liable to erode neighbouring structures such as the lung, mediastinum, oesophagus, vertebral column or pleura, producing a wide range of symptoms. Sooner or later the thinned fibrous wall may rupture, leading to a sudden massive and fatal haemorrhage. Microscopically, the wall of the aneurysm will consist of an outer layer of fibrous tissue and an inner layer of organizing laminated thrombus. Chronic inflammatory cells are usually present in the adventitia.

Other arterial lesions

Endarteritis obliterans

This is a commonly observed change consisting of concentric fibrous thickening of the arterial intima. The change is seen in those situations where the artery is not required to supply such an abundant blood supply as in the past. Examples are in the post-partum myometrium, in the floor of a chronic peptic ulcer, and in the wall of a chronically inflamed gall bladder. In the last two instances the metabolic activities of the new-formed fibrous tissue are less than the epithelium and smooth muscle it has replaced. This phenomenon protects the patient with a peptic ulcer from having as many massive haemorrhages as he might otherwise have on the occasions when arteries become eroded in the ulcerating process.

Polyarteritis nodosa

The acute arteritis resembles that in the Arthus phenomenon. The disease may develop without any obvious precipitating factor. It is very similar to a hypersensitivity arteritis that develops in response to drugs and infections. Some patients present with an illness similar to rheumatoid arthritis and progress to polyarteritis nodosa. Adult males are affected more commonly than women. The lesions are found most frequently in medium-sized muscular or small arteries in the kidneys, skeletal muscle, heart, liver and gastrointestinal tract. The skin, central nervous system and joints are also commonly involved. In the kidneys, as well as arteritic lesions, there may be involvement of capillaries in the glomerular tuft. Renal failure and hypertension are important complications of this disease. Some patients respond to corticosteroid therapy but many die as a result of renal, cardiac or cerebral damage.

Temporal arteritis

This is a focal inflammatory reaction involving the temporal arteries usually of old people, leading to intractable headache. Other cranial arteries may be affected, one of the more common being that to the eye in which case blindness follows. Microscopically, there is acute inflammation of the arterial wall and fibrosis of the intima. Granulomatous foci containing foreign-body giant cells, polymorphs, lymphocytes and plasma cells develop in relation to the degenerate elastic laminae. The disease may extend to involve other sites including the kidney.

Wegener's granulomatosis

This disease has many features similar to those of polyarteritis nodosa. However, it characteristically involves the respiratory tract with granulomatous arteritis in the nasopharynx and lungs. There is usually renal involvement and other organs may also be affected.

Thromboangiitis obliterans (Buerger's disease)

Besides atheroma, thromboangiitis is another cause of intermittent claudication, occurring in younger people than the former. At the time of symptoms, the artery shows occlusion by a recanalized thrombus which is considered to be the end-result of inflammation of the vessel wall, though no persisting inflammatory reaction can usually be identified. The disease has only rarely been observed in the acute stage. In the chronic stage of the disease the obliterative arterial thrombi may contain giant-cell granulomas. The veins may also be affected and the perivascular fibrosis may spread to include the adjacent nerves. Many consider that thromboangiitis is not an entity but represents the results of atherosclerosis, thrombosis or embolism, alone or in combination.

Other aneurysms

The so-called *dissecting aneurysm* of the aorta consists of a splitting of the media by blood driven in from the lumen through a breach in the intima. The blood may track back into the pericardium leading to cardiac tamponade, or forward down the aorta, eventually re-entering the iliac branches or escaping through the adventitia to produce torrential bleeding. The dissection arises because of cystic accumulation of mucopolysaccharides in the media (cystic medial necrosis) which weakens the wall. This may result from a congenital abnormality of collagen (Marfan's syndrome) or follow hypertension. It may also be associated with coarctation of the aorta. *Congenital or 'berry' aneurysms* may develop at the junctions of the main arteries in and around the circle of Willis at the base of the brain, as a result of congenital structural defects in the arterial walls. Rupture of such an aneurysm is the basis for subarachnoid haemorrhage. They may also be associated with hypertension and polycystic kidneys. *Mycotic* aneurysms are usually small and arise as a result of bacterial infection of the arterial wall, often as a complication of bacterial endocarditis.

Veins

The superficial veins of the legs of older people are liable, through valvular incompetence, to become dilated and tortuous. Such *varicose veins*, which are very common, show hypertrophy of the muscle in the media in response to the increased hydrostatic pressure. Thrombi sometimes form in them, but they more usually give rise to symptoms through the production of eczema or even ulceration of the overlying and undernourished skin.

Thrombi develop very commonly in the deeper veins of the leg, and are associated with the complication of pulmonary emboli (see p. 50). Thrombi may form in bacteria-infected veins, but this is a much less frequent clinical problem. *Thrombophlebitis migrans* is a disease which may complicate carcinoma, particulary of the pancreas. The vein is occluded by thrombus and the wall infiltrated by inflammatory cells.

Lymphatics

Acute lymphangitis is best known in the form of the thin red line which may be seen in the skin adjacent to an acutely infected focus. *Local obstruction of lymphatics* produces lymphoedema of the part normally drained. The most likely clinical examples occur when the vessels are obliterated by malignant disease (e.g. the peau d'orange in carcinoma of the breast), after radiotherapy (e.g. lymphoedema of the arm following irradiation of the breast and axilla for carcinoma), or as a result of congenital absence of lymphatics (Milroy's disease). In the Tropics, infestation of the lymphatics by a filarial parasite is very liable to produce lymphoedema, especially of the legs and scrotum. The chronic lymphoedema so produced gives rise to elephantiasis of the affected part.

Tumours of blood vessels

Angiomas, arising either from blood or lymph capillaries, are common in the skin. They may consist either of capillary vessels or of larger blood spaces—cavernous haemangiomas which give the 'port wine stain'. The latter, when occurring on the head, may be associated with similar dilated vascular spaces in the underlying bone, meninges and brain. Cavernous lymphangiomas in the neck are called cystic hygromas.

Glomus tumours occur mainly in the skin of the hands. They are small but very painful and microscopically can be seen to consist of capillaries surrounded by uniform sheets of glomus cells which normally are found surrounding the endothelium in specialized structures referred to as glomus organs. These tumours should not be confused with tumours of the jugular bulb (*glomus jugulare*) or *carotid body* or similar tumours of the aortic arch and elsewhere. They arise from specialized chemoreceptor cells in the vessel wall and are related to tumours of the adrenal gland and sympathetic chain (phaeochromocytoma) which produce catecholamines.

Angiosarcomas are rare. Those arising from blood vessels can be divided into tumours of endothelial origin and those of pericyte origin. The latter sometimes resemble smooth muscle tumours, e.g. uterine 'fibroids'. Lymphangiosarcomas are found following chronic lymphatic obstruction. Angiosarcomas are highly malignant tumours, freely metastasizing as may be assumed from their close relationship with the lumina of vessels. Angiosarcomas of the liver are associated with industrial exposure to vinyl chloride monomer.

Kaposi's sarcoma is usually classified with angiosarcomas but the cell of origin is uncertain. It occurs in parts of Central Europe and Africa, most commonly in adult males. Multiple tumours in the skin and viscera consist of small blood vessels and spindle cells which appear sarcomatous. Interest has been stimulated recently by the association of acquired immune deficiency syndrome (AIDS) in male homosexuals with Kaposi's sarcoma. A possible viral aetiology (human T-cell lymphoma virus — HTLV) has been suggested for AIDS.

14

The Respiratory System

The lungs

It is in the post-mortem room rather than the operating theatre that pathological abnormalities in the lungs are most commonly observed. Before discussing individual diseases, certain changes will first be described which may arise from more than one cause. The normal lung is spongy and dry when cut. In the infant and the country dweller it is mottled pinkish grey in colour, whereas that of the adult town-dweller is greyish black, because of the considerable amount of soot which the lung accumulates from the atmosphere.

Congestion

The acutely congested lung is dark purplish red, and when cut and compressed will exude more blood than normal. Common causes of acute congestion are left ventricular failure and acute inflammation. The lung of chronic venous congestion due to mitral stenosis tends to be tougher than normal, and the cut surface presents a lighter chocolate-brown colour. Microscopically the alveolar capillaries of congested lungs are conspicuous because they are filled with blood. In chronic congestion there are in addition an abundance of histiocytes containing haemosiderin in the alveolar lumina ('heart-failure cells').

Oedema

Pulmonary oedema makes the lung more solid than normal macroscopically, and on palpation transmits the sensation given by a wet sponge. The cut surface exudes abundant clear fluid on compression. Microscopically the alveolar lumina are filled with a clear, lightly eosinophilic exudate. Common causes are acute left ventricular failure, early acute infection, following cerebral injury or after inhalation of a chemical irritant. In 'uraemic lung', the fluid has a higher protein content than in simple oedema and it does not flow as easily from the cut surfaces.

Fibrosis

Fibrosis of the lung can result from a wide range of precipitating factors.

Infective causes are unresolved pneumonias, tuberculosis, chronic bronchitis and bronchiectasis. It may result from malignant disease, sarcoidosis and excessive radiotherapy. It is a dominant feature in the occupational hazard of pneumoconiosis when it follows inhalation of irritant dusts such as silica and asbestos (silicosis, asbestosis). It may occur focally or be diffusely distributed, and the naked-eye picture is one of firm pale-grey plaques or streaks.

Collapse

Collapse of lung occurs when the air normally contained in the alveoli becomes absorbed and is not replaced through respiration. As might be expected, the volume of the collapsed lung is less than normal so that the pleural surface becomes wrinkled. The lung is more solid than normal and of uniform deep purple-grey (or 'slaty') colour. Collapse arises as a result of obstruction of the bronchial tree supplying the area, the commonest cause of the obstruction being undrained bronchial secretion, but others are neoplasms and inhaled foreign bodies. It will also result through compression by an expanded pleural cavity as in effusion or pneumothorax. 'Massive collapse' is the name given to the acute emergency liable to arise after abdominal operations, but which is precipitated by the common cause, undrained bronchial secretions.

Atelectasis

This is the state of a lung when it has never been expanded by air, and is therefore a phenomenon of stillbirth or the neonatal period. Birth injuries to the brain are considered to play an important part in its production; aspirated amniotic fluid may be contributory. As might be expected, the general appearance is that of collapse.

Hyaline membrane disease

This condition occurs in the newborn. It derives its name from the layer of protein exudate which is found in the respiratory bronchioles and alveolar ducts. This exudate stains with eosin and on microscopy is described as a hyaline membrane. It develops particularly in premature infants, those born by Caesarian section and in children of diabetic mothers; the baby develops respiratory distress some hours or days after birth. These infants often die and the lungs are found to be collapsed and airless, with hyaline membrane seen on microscopy. It is believed to be due to a lack of surfactant, a surface-tension-lowering substance produced by type II pneumocytes. In the absence of surfactant, lung expansion is more difficult; hypoxia ensues, leading to changes in permeability of the alveolar capillaries which allows the development of the exudate, and this exacerbates the condition. Similar hyaline membranes can be found in adults in such conditions as uraemia and viral pneumonia, but they are not usually as extensive.

Pneumonia

Definition

Pneumonia can be defined as the filling of the air spaces of the lung with inflammatory exudate. The exudate may involve the whole or part of a lobe. In the former instance, it is termed *lobar pneumonia*. If the consolidated alveoli are clustered round the terminal portions of the bronchial tree, the inflammation is termed *bronchopneumonia*. These two patterns of disease are not specific for any particular organism.

Aetiology

Pneumonia can be a primary inflammation of the lung substance or it can be secondary to another disease process such as carcinoma or chronic bronchitis. The infecting organism is frequently undetermined but is usually bacterial or viral, or sometimes due to other agents. *Streptococcus pneumoniae* and *Haemophilus influenzae* are the commonest bacterial causes, but *Klebsiella* and *Staphylococcus* are not rare. *Mycobacterium tuberculosis* is now a rare cause of bronchopneumonia in Britain. Adenoviruses, respiratory syncytial virus, Coxsackie and Echoviruses as well as influenza virus can all cause pneumonia. *Legionella pneumophila* is a recently recognized cause of pneumonia, resulting in legionnaire's disease. In the immunocompromised host, opportunistic organisms such as *Pneumocystis carinii* or fungi may cause pneumonia. Many factors which impair the defences of the lung play a part in the development of pneumonia.

Pathology

Lobar pneumonia is not now commonly seen in the post-mortem room. It virtually never follows the old-fashioned dramatic clinical picture, but tends to be the somewhat surprising finding in an old person, who may well have been afebrile and, perhaps, discovered unconscious at his or her home. Macroscopically four stages are recognized. The first is one of *congestion* and is followed by an exudative phase in which the lung is red and solid (*red hepatization*). In the third stage the lung is paler grey and drier (*grey hepatization*). In the patient who recovers, the lung returns to its normal state (*resolution*). Microscopically, in the first stage there is congestion of the alveolar capillaries and this is followed by exudation of red cells, fibrin and neutrophil polymorphs into the alveoli. In the stage of grey hepatization the alveolar capillaries are collapsed and bloodless, the exudate now consisting mainly of neutrophil polymorphs. During resolution the alveolar exudate liquefies, and part is coughed up and part absorbed.

Complications sometimes follow. The inflammatory reaction usually spreads to the pleural surface so that pleurisy occurs. This may cause a pleural effusion which is rich in protein and fibrin and has the characteristics of an exudate. There may be a purulent exudate giving an empyema. Infection may spread to give pericarditis. The lung parenchyma may break down to form a lung abscess. This is commoner with some types of pneumococci and staphylococci. Instead of resolution of the pneumonic exudate, this may become organized to form a carnified or fibrotic lung.

Bronchopneumonia is a much commoner picture in the post-mortem room. Macroscopically, the involved lung appears congested and oedematous, and on palpation may feel lumpy. When the cut surface is examined, the diagnostic feature is a cluster of minute pale solid nodules surrounding small bronchi or bronchioles. Histologically, the bronchiolar wall is inflamed and its lumen filled with polymorphs; the adjacent alveoli show similar changes. The more peripheral alveoli are congested and oedematous, the inflammatory reaction here being at an earlier stage of evolution. With severe infections, adjacent solid areas coalesce to produce an incomplete lobar pattern. Bronchopneumonia always causes some destruction of the lung parenchyma. In old people already suffering from chronic lung disease, this additional destruction further reduces the pulmonary reserve.

Suppurative bronchopneumonia, in which multiple abscesses form in the consolidated areas, is a common picture in staphylococcal infection, a disease of considerable gravity.

The commonest picture of pneumonia seen at the present time consists of the non-specific combination of congestion and oedema; this is because of the antibiotic therapy which is practically invariably given. The disease which used to be referred to as primary atypical virus pneumonia is now recognized as being caused by a *Mycoplasma* and not a virus. It is frequently associated with the presence of cold agglutinins in the blood and may be suspected histologically if the exudate in the alveolar wall consists predominantly of histiocytes and lymphocytes rather than polymorphs.

Influenza

This infection is a common winter illness but every few years it occurs as a pandemic. Certain strains of the virus are more pathogenic than others and cause serious disease with a high mortality, particularly in the elderly and very young. At post-mortem the lungs are congested and oedematous with areas of haemorrhage. The trachea and major bronchi show violaceous congestion and contain thin haemorrhagic secretion.

Microscopically there is mononuclear cell infiltration of the alveolar septa and walls of the larger air passages. The alveolar lumen may contain haemorrhagic oedema but polymorphs are usually scanty, unless there is a secondary bacterial infection giving bronchopneumonia.

Lipid pneumonia is either exogenous or endogenous. Exogenous lipid pneumonia is caused by the inhalation of lipid, the two common sources being cod-liver oil and oily nasal drops. Endogenous lipid pneumonia may be found distal to a bronchial obstruction and the lipid comes from the lipoprotein in cell membranes being broken down and ingested by histiocytes.

Chronic bronchitis and emphysema

These two diseases are considered together because they are so commonly associated, and are the basis of a considerable morbidity among the older section of the population in Britain. Epidemiological studies have shown a strong association with smoking.

The clinical yardstick for *chronic bronchitis* is the production of an excessive amount of sputum on most days for three months of the year for two successive years. The constant pathological change is an increased thickness of the glands of the bronchi with a preponderance of mucus-secreting cells. The ratio of gland to wall thickness (the Reid index) is greater than 35% in chronic bronchitis. Squamous metaplasia of the surface epithelium is also seen. The bronchial walls are infiltrated by inflammatory cells during acute episodes of infection, but do not usually become further damaged. Chronic bronchitis produces airways obstruction by increased production of viscid mucus, predisposes to infection and leads to the development of emphysema.

Emphysema may be defined as the lung condition in which there is an increase beyond the normal in the size of the air spaces distal to the terminal bronchiole, with dilatation and destruction of their walls. The classification of emphysema depends mainly on the distribution of dilated air spaces within the secondary lung lobule. *Centrilobular emphysema* shows dilatation or destruction of respiratory bronchioles, whereas *panacinar (panlobular)* emphysema shows this dilatation throughout the lobule. A rare variety of emphysema is confined to the paraseptal region of the lobule. Adjacent to scars, the emphysema is unrelated to the lobule and is related only to the scarring—*focal emphysema*.

Centrilobular emphysema is frequently found in association with chronic bronchitis. It is suggested that the recurrent attacks of bronchiolitis damage the wall of the bronchiole and adjacent alveoli, causing scarring around the bronchiole with subsequent compensatory dilatation of the neighbouring respiratory bronchioles and alveoli. This dilatation results in an increase in the dead space of the lung and a decreased area for exchange of gases. Pulmonary hypertension develops with right ventricular hypertrophy leading to cor pulmonale. The pulmonary arteries become atheromatous. The cause of this pulmonary hypertension is complex. It is due mainly to spasm of the small arteries caused by hypoxia as they cross the dilated air spaces in the centre of the lobule, and in part to opening up of anastomoses between the pulmonary arteries and bronchial arteries which contain blood at systemic blood pressure. Destruction of lung tissue also increases the resistance of the pulmonary vascular bed. Eventually the heart fails and chronic venous congestion develops. Panacinar emphysema is less frequently associated with chronic bronchitis, and although the amount of lung damage may appear greater, pulmonary hypertension is less noticeable. However, as the total area for gas exchange is reduced, patients are dyspnoeic.

There are two clinical types of patients with pulmonary emphysema. One, caricatured as the 'blue bloater', has central cyanosis and signs of cor pulmonale, with a high arterial P_{CO_2} and low P_{O_2}. The 'pink puffer' lacks central cyanosis and cor pulmonale but breathes rapidly and, under normal circumstances, maintains his normal blood gas values. These are ends of a spectrum and many patients do not fall into either category. The reasons for the different clinical presentations are not always clear.

Macroscopically, emphysema may be inconspicuous unless the lung is fixed inflated. Sometimes the emphysema develops into polypoid projections near the surface, called bullae. These are liable to perforate, leading to escape of air into the pleural cavity—pneumothorax.

Bronchial asthma

This is a functional condition characterized by recurrent episodes of restriction of airflow due to temporary narrowing of small air passages. There are two main types. *Atopic* (extrinsic) *asthma* usually starts in childhood; there is often demonstrable allergy to an extrinsic antigen such as pollen or house dust mite. These patients often have an atopic family history and type I hypersensitivity plays a part in the development of attacks. *Non-atopic* (intrinsic) *asthma* occurs in older people lacking histories of eczema or asthma in the family; no hypersensitivity to an allergen is demonstrable.

Attacks usually remit with treatment. When death occurs, the lungs are found to be distended, the small airways are plugged with mucus, and the bronchial mucosa is congested, oedematous and shows an eosinophil infiltrate; the bronchial smooth muscle may be thicker than normal. Should an atopic asthmatic die between attacks for unrelated reasons, it is usually difficult to demonstrate any structural lesion in the lung.

Pneumoconioses

These lung diseases are caused by the inhalation of dust, usually as an industrial hazard. They may be divided into two groups: those caused by mineral dusts, and those caused by organic dusts, the latter causing damage to the lung largely through an immunological reaction (extrinsic allergic alveolitis). The former mineral dust disease can be further subdivided into those caused by fibrogenic and non-fibrogenic dusts.

Silicosis is due to the inhalation of silica dust, most commonly in coal mines or quarries where stone containing silica has to be cut. The larger particles are removed by the action of cilia in the major air passages, but the particles of less than 3 μm enter the alveoli where they are ingested by macrophages. These macrophages enter lymphatics which they block, and thus cause a fibrous reaction. Surrounding this there is focal emphysema. These patients also have a high incidence of tuberculosis which may contribute to the lung scarring.

Anthracosis. Carbon does not itself cause fibrosis, but in mines the carbon of coal often contains small quantities of silica. The carbon inhaled by city dwellers appears to be inert in the lung.

Asbestosis is caused by the inhalation of asbestos (magnesium silicate) in the manufacture of insulating material and in industries concerned with pipe lagging and brake lining. It is an important cause of pulmonary fibrosis, and also causes an increased incidence of carcinoma of the lung and mesothelioma of the pleura. It is particularly blue asbestos (crocidolite) which causes this reaction, but other forms may also do so. It is now thought that the physical properties of the needle-shaped crystals play an important part in this reaction.

Extrinsic allergic alveolitis

Organic dusts may cause lung disease via a type III hypersensitivity reaction. The best-known example is *farmer's lung* in which inhalation of the thermophilic *Micropolyspora faeni* from mouldy hay results in pulmonary damage in some individuals. The patients affected are those who produce high levels of precipitating antibody in the serum. An attack of breathlessness occurs several hours after exposure to the dust. Inhaled antigens combine with serum antibody in the alveolar wall, and the immune complexes so formed activate complement; mediators are released which stimulate an acute inflammatory process. Repeated exposure leads to giant-cell granuloma formation—presumably a cell-mediated (type IV) reaction—and ultimately to pulmonary fibrosis with all its complications. Other diseases such as bird fancier's lung (bird droppings), mushroom worker's lung (compost), and bagassosis (sugar-cane residue) give very similar clinical pictures but are caused by different antigens.

Bronchiectasis

Bronchiectasis is a condition in which the bronchi become dilated either in cylindrical or saccular form. The disease is most common in the lower lobe bronchi and is associated with the production of abundant foul sputum, which cannot be drained away as effectively as normal. Microscopically, the wall of the dilated bronchus is usually heavily infiltrated with chronic inflammatory cells and the muscular coat appears thinned. There is destruction of cartilage and metaplasia of the lining epithelium to a stratified squamous pattern. Ulceration of the mucous membrane will take place in the later stages, and there will be a varying degree of collapse and fibrosis of the surrounding lung. Bronchiectasis is considered to be due to: (1) weakening of the supporting tissue of the bronchial wall by inflammation, (2) contraction of the surrounding fibrous tissue, and (3) increased pull by inspiration as a result of the collapse of the surrounding lung. It is usually a sequel to severe acute infections, such as measles and whooping cough in the earlier years. There is often associated nasal sinusitis and the drainage of the infected secretion into the lungs during sleep may cause other cases. The disease is becoming less common nowadays, probably as a result of the more effective treatment by antibiotics. Lung abscesses, metastatic abscesses, especially in the brain, and amyloid disease are well-recognized complications.

Tuberculosis

Pulmonary tuberculosis in Britain has decreased dramatically in prevalence over the last 40 years. This is partly due to the availability of adequate treatment and partly to the higher standard of living of the population. It is by no means extinct, however, and remains a cause of death particularly in the elderly and those in poor social conditions. The other major group in whom it is seen is young immigrants to the UK, often presenting with a pyrexia of unknown origin.

The primary infection leads to the development of a 'Ghon focus', which is usually midzonal and subpleural in situation. It consists of the characteristic granulomatous inflammatory reaction which may become caseous; the hilar lymph nodes draining the focus may also become involved. The Ghon focus heals to form a fibrous or calcified nodule in the vast majority of cases. With re-infection, the classical post-primary lesion develops at the apex of one or both lungs, consisting at first of a localized pneumonic consolidation before the characteristic tubercles develop. This again heals in the great majority of people often without symptoms, to produce the sometimes calcified apical scars so commonly seen in the lungs of people in civilized communities. In some individuals, however, the disease will spread and become clinically evident. The caseation in individual tubercles coalesces and the softened lung tissue may be removed by expectoration so that a cavity develops. The lung in the untreated case becomes increasingly disorganized and fibrosed with continued spread of the infection, usually by way of the lymphatics. The state of fibrocaseous tuberculosis eventually results, which is very much more difficult to cure, and which in fact may lead to death of the patient through progressive deterioration of respiratory reserve. The pleura may become involved in the chronic progression of the disease with the result that fibrous adhesions develop, or sometimes bronchopleural fistula forms, leading to pneumothorax and tuberculous empyema. The progression of the disease may become more active as a result of rupture of infected material into a bronchus and spread therefrom into the related alveoli, leading to pneumonia which in its most active form is a confluent bronchopneumonia (caseous pneumonia or 'galloping consumption').

Another common presentation of respiratory tuberculosis in the early post-primary phase is a pleural effusion. The fluid is clear and may be abundant, containing lymphocytes from which tubercle bacilli can sometimes be cultured. The effusion usually subsides completely, even without specific therapy, leaving no radiological evidence of underlying pulmonary infection. Biopsy and endoscopy studies have shown, however, that the affected pleura contains a number of tubercles. The amount of effusion and the rapidity with which it forms suggest that the fluid exudes from much of the pleural surface, probably as a manifestation of the hypersensitive state.

The common complication of pulmonary tuberculosis is spread of the infection to elsewhere in the body. A primary focus, particularly that in a hilar lymph node, is liable to erode into a blood vessel, and the flooding of tubercule bacilli into organs, particularly when resistance is low, leads to the formation of *miliary tuberculosis*. This serious event was an important cause of death in children in pre-antibiotic days because of the development of tuberculous meningitis. Tubercle bacilli draining into the thoracic duct may give rise to miliary tuberculosis in the lungs. Spread from a tuberculous cavity via the major air passages may involve the intestinal tract as a result of swallowed sputum, leading to tuberculous ulcers of the bowel, ileocaecal 'hyperplastic' tuberculosis or fistula-in-ano. Renal tuberculosis is a blood-borne infection, usually starting from an active pulmonary lesion. Amyloidosis is a complication liable to develop in cases of long-standing pulmonary tuberculosis. The pulmonary fibrosis associated particularly with the secondary infection is liable to cause focal emphysema and bronchiectasis. Carcinomas sometimes arise in old tuberculous scars following metaplasia of alveolar epithelium at the periphery of the scar.

Sarcoidosis

The lesion of a sarcoid reaction is similar to a tubercle except that caseation does not occur and acid-fast bacilli cannot be demonstrated. The majority of cases of sarcoidosis show diffuse pulmonary infiltration which may scar to give a 'honeycomb lung'. Lymph nodes, spleen, liver, skin, uveal tract, salivary and lacrimal glands are all commonly involved. There may be bone lesions in the hands similar to those of hyperparathyroidism and these may be accompanied by a raised serum calcium and nephrocalcinosis. A few cases eventually show features of tuberculosis, but in the majority the aetiology remains obscure. In addition to the characteristic histological changes, the diagnosis may be confirmed by a positive *Kveim test*. This test depends on the intradermal injection of a phenolized extract of a sarcoid spleen with the development of a characteristic sarcoid reaction six weeks later. A local sarcoid reaction is sometimes seen in lymph nodes draining malignant lesions, or in the lungs, skin and lymph nodes in berylliosis, but these cases do not have a positive Kveim test and they should not be diagnosed as sarcoidosis.

Carcinoma of bronchus

Bronchial carcinoma is a disease of considerable importance because it is now the commonest fatal cancer, and in Britain in men aged 45–64 the numbers of deaths from lung cancer are now equal to those from all other forms of cancer together. It enters into the differential diagnosis of most of the persistent respiratory ailments, and of a good many others presenting outside this system. Careful epidemiological studies have shown that the way is open to diminish, and perhaps largely obliterate, its incidence. These investigations have shown beyond any reasonable doubt that the incidence of this cancer parallels the incidence of cigarette smoking, and that the risk is greatest among the heaviest smokers. Cigarette smoke contains both cancer initiators and cancer promoters. The former include polycyclic aromatic hydrocarbons and the latter phenols, fatty acid esters and free fatty acids. Laboratory animals have developed lung cancer after being trained to inhale cigarette smoke. In man the risk of developing lung cancer is increased approximately thirty-fold for those smoking 30 cigarettes per day.

Macroscopic appearance

The macroscopic picture of carcinoma of the bronchus varies extremely widely, as any regular visitor to the post-mortem room knows. The tumour may start anywhere in the bronchial tree and in any lobe. It is commoner in the larger primary divisions of the bronchi than elsewhere. The tumour may be so small that meticulous dissection by an experienced pathologist is necessary to reveal it; on the other hand, it may be so extensive as to involve much of the lung, spreading even to cover the whole of the pleural surface. The frequency of pleural involvement is indicated by the frequency of pleural effusion as a presenting symptom, from which malignant cells may be identified in a cytological specimen. The tumour may consist merely of a roughening of the bronchial surface, which can be associated with a considerable infiltration of the surrounding lung tissue, or it may cause occlusion of the bronchial lumen, either by growing into it as a polypoid tumour, or by cicatrizing it by growing round in the wall. The less common peripherally situated tumours often appear as spherical masses, with which no communication with a bronchus can be clearly demonstrated. Some of these arise in a fibrous scar in the lung, e.g. at the site of healed tuberculosis. These scars frequently contain atypical bronchiolar–alveolar cells which are believed to be the starting point of such tumours. On section, the tumour most commonly presents a pale-grey or brown cut surface. A wide variety of secondary changes can occur in the lung drained by the affected bronchus. It can be congested, oedematous, consolidated, emphysematous, collapsed or bronchiectatic, and more than one feature can be present at the same time. The tumour may cavitate as a result of necrosis so that fluid levels may be seen radiologically.

Microscopic appearance

The commonest type is a *squamous cell carcinoma* (40–60%) which arises from abnormal metaplastic squamous epithelium in the bronchi. *Adenocarcinoma* (about 10%) is the least common type, arising peripherally, sometimes associated with scars. There are two forms of *anaplastic carcinoma*—the *large cell type* (10–15%) which may resemble squamous carcinoma but lacks keratin or prickles, and the *small or oat cell type* (20–30%). It is widely believed that the oat cell carcinoma arises from cells of the diffuse endocrine system in the bronchial mucosa and is therefore a highly malignant counterpart of the carcinoid tumour.

Spread

The different patterns of spread are legion. A minute tumour may be associated with many and widespread metastases. A large tumour infiltrating locally may show few or no secondary growths. The direct spread is commonly into the hilum and on into the mediastinum, with the result that the great vessels may become encased or compressed, the recurrent laryngeal nerve infiltrated, and the pericardium widely permeated. A tumour arising arising near the apex of the lung may give rise to Pancoast's syndrome which consists of symptoms due to brachial plexus and cervical sympathetic infiltration. Lymph node metastases are common and may be distant, though those at the hilum, in the neck, and axilla, are most commonly involved. The hilar node enlargement may be considerable and produce mediastinal obstructive symptoms. As the lung is a vascular structure in immediate communication with the systemic circulation, it is not surprising that blood-borne metastases are common and may be widespread. Cutaneous metastases, for example, are often the first diagnostic sign that the tumour exists in a patient. Cerebral metastases are the commonest malignant tumours in that tissue. The bronchus is one of the likely primary sites from which carcinoma may produce osteolytic skeletal metastases. The liver is very frequently infiltrated, and the tumour appears to have a predilection to metastasize to the adrenal glands.

Systemic manifestations

Besides producing sometimes unexpected symptoms and signs by way of metastases, bronchial carcinoma can also be responsible for other syndromes for which the presence of tumour cannot be directly implicated. Endocrinological syndromes are particularly associated with oat cell carcinoma. These include: (1) Cushing's syndrome with hyperplasia of the adrenal cortex, and (2) inappropriate secretion of antidiuretic hormone leading to hyponatraemia. Neurological syndromes include a peripheral neuromyopathy and cerebellar degeneration. Other syndromes include dermatomyositis, hypertrophic pulmonary osteoarthropathy and thrombophlebitis migrans. Squamous cell carcinoma may be associated with hypercalcaemia, simulating hyperparathyroidism.

Bronchial adenoma

These tumours occur earlier in life and there is not the same discrepancy in sex incidence as there is in bronchial carcinomas. They appear in the larger bronchi as polypoid growths, but the great bulk of the tumour is locally infiltrative in the bronchial wall. Histologically, two patterns are found, carcinoid tumours and cylindromas. The former resemble the carcinoid tumour of the alimentary tract and a few produce the carcinoid syndrome (flushing, cyanosis, diarrhoea and occasionally pulmonary stenosis) with an increased urinary excretion of 5-hydroxyindoleacetic acid (5-HIAA). Cylindromas resemble salivary gland tumours. Both types occasionally metastasize and should therefore be regarded as carcinomas, though they are less aggressive than bronchial carcinoma.

Pulmonary hamartoma

These tumour-like malformations are usually detected on routine chest x-ray, where they are seen as rounded shadows in the lung field. They consist of abundant bronchial cartilage intimately mixed with glandular epithelium—hence their alternative name of adenochondroma. They are benign.

The larynx and trachea

Acute infection of the larynx frequently occurs as part of an upper respiratory infection. The development of the inflammatory reaction may so interfere with the normal function of the vocal cord that hoarseness results. An important acute infection that used to occur in

Britain and still remains in other parts of the world is diphtheria. This is characterized by the development of a pseudomembrane consisting of necrotic debris, exudate and fragments of shed epithelium. The exotoxin produced by the organism gives rise to systemic effects on the heart and nervous system. *Tuberculous ulceration* may develop secondarily to spreading pulmonary infection. *Oedema*, from any cause involving the larynx, may produce acute respiratory distress necessitating a tracheotomy (e.g. angioneurotic oedema). Oedematous nodules are common lesions on the vocal cords ('singer's nodes'); they are brought about by constriction of lax mucous membrane by the movements of the cords during talking and singing. Recurrent squamous cell *papillomas* may at times be seen and are probably viral in origin.

Squamous cell carcinomas may develop in the larynx, accounting for rather less than 1% of all malignant tumours in the body. The tumours may be intrinsic, occurring just below, on, or just above the vocal cords, or extrinsic, arising on the epiglottis, aryepiglottic folds or pyriform fossa. They spread by local invasion or lymph node metastases; bloodstream spread is uncommon. The extrinsic tumours spread more readily and therefore have the worse prognosis.

Serious pathological conditions are uncommon in the trachea. It frequently takes part in the inflammation produced by upper respiratory infections; malignant disease is distinctly rare.

15

The Tissues of Head and Neck

The lips

Squamous cell carcinoma of the lip accounts for 1% of all malignant tumours. It is frequently preceded by dysplasia of the epithelium. It is commoner in the older age groups and much more frequent in men than women. There is an increased incidence among pipe smokers and fair-skinned individuals exposed to excessive sun. The tumour occurs particularly on the lower lip, infiltrates locally and ulcerates. Metastases are usually to the submandibular or pre-auricular lymph nodes. The ulcerated tumour is liable to become severely infected.

The tongue

Atrophy of the glossal epithelium, with flattening of papillae and desquamation of the mucocutaneous junction at the angle of the lips (angular stomatitis) occurs in deficiency states of which lack of iron and vitamin B_{12} are important examples. Iron deficiency produces atrophy at the sides first, compared with the total atrophy and inflammatory reaction of vitamin B_{12} deficiency. Intestinal disorders leading to riboflavine and nicotinamide deficiencies, and oral antibiotic therapy, produce similar lesions.

Squamous cell carcinoma of the tongue makes up 1% of all malignant tumours. The incidence is approximately equal between the sexes, and the tumour is commoner among the older age groups. Keratinization of dysplastic epithelium giving white plaques may precede carcinoma developing in the anterior part of the tongue. The tumour spreads in the same way as carcinoma of the lip and shows the same liability to ulceration.

The mouth

Mucus-retention cysts are common, consisting usually of small swellings in the buccal cavity and arising as a result of blockage of the duct of one of the many salivary glands that open into the mouth.

Teeth frequently become carious, and the tooth sockets may be the seat of chronic, sometimes purulent, inflammation producing apical abscesses (gumboils) and pyorrhoea. Infected tooth sockets are believed to be the portal of entry for *Actinomyces israeli*. This organism, causing actinomycosis, sets up an acute inflammatory reaction in the jaw which extends to the overlying skin. The tissue becomes wood-hard and multiple skin sinuses discharge the characteristic 'sulphur granules'. Staining of the buccal mucosa adjacent to teeth is seen in chronic poisoning with heavy metals, e.g. lead. Pigmentation of the oral mucosa may be racial, or genetic, as in the oral pigmentation and intestinal polyposis of Peutz–Jeghers syndrome. Addison's disease may also cause buccal pigmentation.

Dentigerous cysts are squamous epithelial-lined cysts around unerupted teeth, whereas *dental cysts* are squamous epithelial-lined cysts around root abscesses. Sometimes the inflammation produces a local swelling of the gum (an *epulis*) which consists largely of reactive fibrosis to the inflammation.

Infections of the mouth may be viral, bacterial or fungal. Vincent's gingivitis produces acute necrotizing inflammation caused by *Borrelia vincentii* and fusiform bacillus. *Candida albicans* infection (thrush) is a common complication of oral antibiotic therapy; it also occurs in children and debilitated adults. Small white spots contain the mycelial network. The infection may spread into the air passages and oesophagus. The exanthemata show oral lesions, *Koplik's spots* of measles being well known. Lesions are also seen in the mouth in chickenpox and smallpox. Herpes simplex is a common recurring oral viral infection. The virus causes bullous lesions in the oral mucosa; the pathogenesis is similar to that of lesions in the vulva, though usually due to a different strain. *Aphthous ulcers* are small, painful, often recurrent and multiple ulcers which occur in the mouth; their aetiology is still unknown.

Adamantinoma (ameloblastoma) is a tumour arising from the odontogenic epithelium including the enamel organ of the developing tooth. The majority occur in the lower jaw and present as expansile, locally infiltrative tumours. The histological pattern resembles the enamel organ and consists of a reticulum of stellate cells surrounded by columnar or cubical cells. Another tumour which presents as swelling of the jaw is Burkitt's lymphoma which occurs in children in Africa. The gums become diffusely swollen following anti-epileptic drugs and in some cases of leukaemia; *ulcers* may appear in the buccal cavity and throat in leukaemia, and through agranulocytosis. *Squamous cell carcinoma*, apart from that of the tongue, occurs most commonly in the floor of the mouth. Salivary tumours may be seen, especially in the palate, a reminder that numerous small glands exist within the buccal cavity.

The throat

Acute inflammation, with ulceration and deeper extension (quinsy), occurs in the tonsil and at the back of the throat and is usually due to *Streptococcus pyogenes*. Another cause of acute inflammation, diphtheria, is nowadays rare in the UK. *Chronic inflammation* of the tonsil leads to considerable lymphoid hyperplasia, particularly in the young. Glandular fever often presents as a sore throat with lymphadenopathy.

Squamous cell carcinoma is the commonest malignant tumour of tonsil and pharynx; in the latter situation it tends to be poorly differentiated and of relatively poor prognosis. Anaplastic carcinomas in this area are sometimes referred to as *lymphoepitheliomas*. These tumours are most common in the Far East. Often being small, they may be overlooked and present first with lymph node metastases in the neck. Because of the abundant lymphoid tissue in this region, *malignant lymphoma* is only a little less frequent than carcinoma. The natural history is that of malignant lymphoma in general.

The nose and nasal sinuses

This area differs from the mouth and throat in that, being part of the respiratory system, it is lined by ciliated pseudostratified columnar epithelium. Hypersecretion is therefore as prominent a feature of *infection* as it is in the bronchi. This will be obvious to most through experience of that common virus infection, the cold. The mucous membrane also becomes congested, and it is the combination of congestion, hypersecretion, and slowing of ciliary action which is responsible for the stuffiness so typical of the disease. In the later stages, the voluminous water secretion gives way to one which is more scanty, viscid, and purulent, due in part to secondary bacterial infection.

The continued production of secretion and its ineffective drainage through their orifices are responsible for the unpleasantly painful symptoms of acute and chronic *sinusitis*, and treatment, both medical and surgical, is directed towards improving the drainage. Chronic infection causes lymphoid swelling to occur at the back of the nose in the young, producing the well-known obstructive lesion of *adenoids*.

Inflammatory changes also result from *hay fever* or allergic rhinitis, and eosinophils are prominent in the inflammatory exudate. A moderately common late result of any one of the above types of inflammation, or a combination of them, is the development of nasal polyps, which tend to be recurrent. They consist of oedematous and inflamed submucosa covered by normal epithelium. Nasal papillomas differ from inflammatory polyps in that they are covered by transitional epithelium, tend to recur but rarely give rise to invasive tumours (Ringertz tumours). *Nose bleeds* are common phenomena, which are usually of trivial importance, but which on occasions may be so persistent and recurrent that serious anaemia develops. Most arise through congestion following virus infection, some follow trauma, others occur in hypertensive patients and those with blood diseases. A few arise through vascular abnormalities (telangiectases).

Carcinoma is the commonest malignant disease here, as elsewhere in the oronasopharynx. It is commoner in Chinese and also has a higher incidence in workers in the wood and nickel industries. The cell type of the carcinoma varies: some are squamous, some are straightforward adenocarcinomas, and others are salivary tumours. Lymphoepitheliomas occur here as in the tonsil. Malignant lymphomas are not rare. Malignant tumours here tend to have a relatively poor prognosis, because of the inaccessibility for complete surgical excision. *Wegener's granulomatosis* is a form of systemic vasculitis similar to polyarteritis nodosa, with small vessels involved in the nasopharynx, the lung and kidney. Giant cell granulomas are often present. The disease has a poor prognosis.

The ear

The *pinna* undergoes the same pathological changes as the skin generally. The *external auditory meatus* is relatively free of common pathological lesions apart from superficial infections. The *eardrum* may perforate after the exudates from secondarily infected virus inflammations, such as the common cold, extend to and accumulate in the middle ear causing distension of the drum. If the infection does not subside quickly afterwards, the persisting sinus may be accompanied by the formation of granulomatous aural polyps (acute and chronic otitis media). *Cholesteatoma* is not a true tumour, but consists of a granulomatous reaction containing squamous epithelium, keratin and cholesterol crystals resulting from chronic inflammation in the middle ear and mastoid. It gradually erodes the temporal bone.

There are three main causes of *deafness*—chronic otitis media, otosclerosis, and degenerative changes in the auditory nerve. Otitis media causes deafness either because the pharyngotympanic (Eustachian) tube becomes blocked by inflammatory exudate or because the eardrum is badly perforated. Otosclerosis is a condition in which the oval window of the bony labyrinth becomes first increasingly vascular, and then transformed to a more spongy bone. Deafness arises when this process, which is of unknown aetiology, extends on to the fibrous annular ligament of the stapes which fits into the window. Degeneration of the auditory nerve is most likely to follow an acute viral infection, such as measles.

The eye

The eye can become disorganized and inflamed as a result of *trauma*. It has long been known that if one eye is damaged, there is a risk of serious destructive inflammation arising in the other one (sympathetic ophthalmia). It is probable that this unwelcome complication has an autoimmune reaction as its basis.

Two primary *malignant tumours* are liable to arise within the eye, with approximately equal frequency. Malignant melanoma is the one more likely to develop in adults of the older age group, arising most frequently in the choroid and detaching the retina over it as it grows. The tumour is liable to spread by way of the bloodstream and is a well-known cause of the appearance of delayed metastases, the liver being frequently thus involved. Retinoblastoma is the tumour which is likely to arise in early life. Most such tumours arise sporadically but some are undoubtedly hereditary. The tumour spreads preferentially along the optic nerve into the brain but may metastasize distantly outside the central nervous system.

Cataract is an opacity of the lens and may be predominantly peripheral or central. Common causes of cataract are senility, trauma, diabetes and congenital defects which may be due to rubella infection during intrauterine life. Diabetes, in addition to causing cataracts, also results in characteristic retinal capillary microaneurysms visible through an ophthalmoscope. Haemorrhages from these aneurysms are associated with vascular proliferation extending into the vitreous and causing retinal detachment—*retinitis proliferans*. *Retrolental fibroplasia* is a condition found in premature babies exposed to an oxygen concentration of more than 40%. It is caused by retinal vascular proliferation extending into the vitreous with condensation of this tissue behind the lens. *Toxoplasmosis* is an infection which is becoming recognized as a cause of choroidoretinitis and may be a congenital infection or acquired in later life.

The *conjunctiva* is liable to many of the pathological changes which affect squamous epithelium elsewhere. Conjunctivitis is the commonest disease to occur and is due to trauma or infection. In the latter case viruses, e.g. adenovirus, are more frequent causal agents than bacteria. An important chlamydial infection in the Tropics is *trachoma*, which results in a heavy lymphocytic infiltration leading to epithelial proliferation. There is vascularization of the cornea and much scarring leading to blindness.

The *orbit* may be the seat of pathological changes which reveal themselves through the eye being pushed forward (proptosis or exophthalmia). This is a well-known complication of hyperthyroidism and it is due to connective tissue oedema. Proptosis can also be produced by malignant tumours, either primary or secondary, occurring in the orbital bones, paranasal air sinuses, orbital fat or optic nerve. Proptosis may be caused by a chronic fibrosing inflammatory process, called pseudo-tumour of the orbit, of unknown aetiology.

The subcutaneous tissues of the neck

The salivary glands

Mumps is a virus infection to which the salivary glands, especially the parotid, are susceptible. As most cases of mumps recover, little is known of the pathological change in this disease, which will also at times infect other tissues in the body, e.g. the pancreas, the testes and the brain. *Suppurative bacterial infection* may occur chiefly in the parotid gland, as a complication of other severe diseases, especially of the gastrointestinal tract. Chronic inflammation and atrophy of the salivary glands may follow obstruction of the main duct by a *calculus*. Much of the epithelial tissue then becomes atrophic and replaced by fat and fibrous tissue. *Sjögren's syndrome* is a cause of salivary gland enlargement. It occurs particularly in middle-aged women and is associated with a dry mouth, dry eyes and rheumatoid arthritis. The salivary and lacrimal glands become infiltrated by lymphocytes and there is atrophy of the epithelium. *Mikulicz's syndrome* is a term used to describe salivary and lacrimal gland enlargement due to a variety of causes including sarcoidosis, tuberculosis, malignant lymphoma and leukaemia.

Salivary gland tumours

These tumours occur predominantly in the parotid gland, the submandibular gland being the next commonest site. Tumours in the sublingual and minor salivary glands in the mouth are uncommon. By far the commonest tumour is the *pleomorphic adenoma* which occurs mainly in the parotid and is sometimes called a *mixed parotid tumour*. It is a lobulated tumour, often poorly encapsulated so that, after attempted excision, tumour remnants are left and give rise to recurrences. The tumour may be firm and glistening or mucoid. It consists of glandular and squamous epithelium in a mucoid stroma resembling cartilage, hence the term 'mixed tumour'. The connective tissue seems to be produced by the myoepithelial cells which form part of the tumour. Rarely, these tumours may become malignant and then develop the features of an adenocarcinoma. Three other varieties of carcinoma are found and these are relatively more common outside the parotid gland. The *cylindroma* or *adenoid cystic carcinoma* consists of cribriform nests of cells separated by strands of hyalinized connective tissue.

The next two tumours are usually of low-grade malignancy: although they infiltrate locally, they rarely metastasize. Some pathologists therefore refer to them as mucoepidermoid and acinic cell *tumours* rather than carcinomas. However, as it is difficult to predict their behaviour, the latter term is used here. *Mucoepidermoid carcinomas* have islands of squamous epithelium containing isolated mucus-secreting cells. *Acinic cell carcinomas* are rare, clear cell or granular cell tumours. These carcinomas tend to be locally recurrent and locally infiltrative, metastasizing rarely to cervical or preauricular lymph nodes.

Warthin's tumour (adenolymphoma) occurs almost exclusively in the parotid gland. It is derived from ductular epithelium and consists of tall columnar epithelium in an abundant lymphoid stroma. These tumours are benign.

Nerve sheath tumours arising on the facial nerve may occur in the parotid gland, but other connective tissue tumours and malignant lymphomas are rare.

Branchial cysts

These congenital cystic structures exist in the lateral aspect of the neck and are usually lined by stratified squamous epithelium surrounded by abundant lymphoid tissue. They are considered to develop from branchial cleft remnants, but this view has its critics.

Thyroglossal cysts

These develop in the midline between the thyroid gland and the back of the tongue in the pathway of the embryonic thyroglossal duct. When in the upper part, they are lined by squamous epithelium; when in the lower, by ciliated columnar epithelium. A few thyroid acini may be present in the wall.

Lymph nodes

Enlarged lymph nodes may frequently be palpated in the neck. Most often the enlargement is due to virus infection (glandular fever, adenovirus) or bacterial infection (*Streptococcus pyogenes*, tuberculosis). Sometimes the enlargement is due to malignant disease, such as malignant lymphoma, or secondary carcinoma.

16

The Alimentary System (I)

The oesophagus

Oesophagitis

Oesophagitis may result from infection, especially monilial infection spreading from the oral cavity. Hot, caustic and corrosive substances may also cause inflammation, ulceration and possibly fibrous stricture. One of the commonest causes of oesophagitis is reflux of gastric contents into the oesophagus and this has come to be appreciated as an important differential diagnosis of myocardial infarction as a cause of substernal pain. It may occur without gross anatomical disorder, but it is especially common when there is a hiatus hernia, i.e. partial herniation of the stomach through the diaphragmatic hiatus. The chronic inflammation may become complicated by ulceration of the mucous membrane, and after a time this may lead to fibrous stricture of the lower end of the oesophagus.

Achalasia

This is a disorder of motility affecting the whole of the oesophagus. Swallowing still promotes muscular activity but peristalsis is lost and the cardiac region remains tonically contracted; as a result, the oesophagus empties incompletely and tends to enlarge. The tonic region does not become greatly hypertrophied. There is evidence of abnormality of the autonomic nerve fibres and ganglia in the muscle coat of the oesophagus, with absence of the normal cholinergic mechanisms of peristalsis.

Oesophageal varices

Oesophageal varices are dilated veins, which connect portal and systemic venous drainage, at the lower end of the oesophagus. They are seen in portal hypertension, which is most often due to cirrhosis. The epithelium overlying varices may ulcerate, leading to rupture of the veins and severe haemorrhage. The diagnosis may be made endoscopically or by radiology. At post-mortem the lesion may be hard to identify because the veins collapse.

Carcinoma

The oesophagus may develop squamous cell carcinoma (almost 3% of malignant tumour deaths). Most arise in the middle third, after which the lower third is more commonly involved than the upper. The disease is liable to arise in the older age groups, with a male preponderance except where it occurs as a complication of the Plummer–Vinson syndrome, which is commoner in women. This syndrome consists of dysphagia, glossitis, hypochlorhydria and iron deficiency anaemia leading to the development of a post-cricoid mucosal web and eventually carcinoma. The carcinoma may project into the lumen. This projection, coupled with the fibrosis of the wall due to the infiltrating carcinoma, leads to obstruction of the lumen which is the basis of the dominant symptom, inability to swallow. The tumour infiltrates through the muscle coat of the oesophagus, and spreads readily into the mediastinum as there is no serosal coat to delay the advancing carcinoma. Mediastinal lymph nodes are commonly involved. Carcinoma of the lower third of the oesophagus frequently spreads via the lymphatics to the lymph nodes on the lesser curve of the stomach. Carcinoma of the upper oesophagus may spread to the cervical lymph nodes. Ulceration into the mediastinum causes a serious inflammatory reaction. Death is usually as a result of inanition, pneumonia following aspiration of food being a contributory factor.

The lower end of the oesophagus, immediately before it enters the saccular stomach, is lined by gastric mucosa. Carcinomas in this area are therefore adenocarcinomas and they are indistinguishable from primary carcinomas in the gastric cardia extending into the lower oesophagus.

Adenocarcinoma may also develop from islands of ectopic gastric mucosa higher in the oesophagus.

Diverticula

A diverticulum is an out-pouching from the lumen. Diverticula may occur all the way along the alimentary tract and be congenital or acquired. When the wall of the diverticulum is composed of mucosa and muscularis propria, it is known as a *true* diverticulum; when the mucosa herniates through the muscularis propria, it is called a *false* diverticulum. Diverticula in the oesophagus are of two types. A *pulsion* diverticulum (false) results from herniation of mucosa in the posterolateral aspect of the hypopharynx between the circular and the oblique fibres of the inferior constrictor muscle of the pharynx. The diverticulum becomes enlarged by swallowing and is filled with undigested food. A *traction* diverticulum (true) may occur in the middle third of the oesophagus due to tuberculosis in mediastinal lymph nodes leading to fibrous contraction of surrounding tissue.

The stomach and duodenum

The study of diffuse lesions of the gastric mucous membrane has for long been hampered because of the extensive autolysis which takes place rapidly after death. Endoscopy and gastric biopsy, added to the study of operative specimens, have made our understanding clearer.

Acute gastritis

Acute gastritis is common in a mild self-limiting form, being produced by the ingestion of various irritants, such as alcohol, aspirin and bacterial toxins (*Staphylococcus, Salmonella*). The mucous membrane shows increased shedding of epithelium and signs of regenerative activity. A small number of inflammatory cells, including polymorphs, may accumulate in the lamina propria. The changes may lead to chronic gastritis.

Chronic gastritis and gastric atrophy

Chronic gastritis is divided into two main types, chronic superficial gastritis and chronic atrophic gastritis. In the former, the thickness of the gastric mucosa is not reduced and the inflammatory reaction is confined to the superficial layers, sparing the deeper glands. This pattern is seen in chronic alcoholics and also shows an increased incidence with age. Chronic atrophic gastritis affects the body of the stomach and causes the mucosa to become thin. The chronic inflammatory reaction extends through the full thickness of the mucosa and there is atrophy of the glandular epithelium. The mucosa may show development of goblet cells in the surface layer of epithelium and Paneth cells in the glands, producing a pattern of epithelium normally found in the intestine and referred to as intestinal metaplasia. This form of gastritis merges imperceptibly into gastric atrophy which is found in patients with Addisonian pernicious anaemia. The loss of oxyntic and parietal cells from the gastric glands results in achlorhydria and absence of intrinsic factor. Antibodies to parietal cells can be demonstrated in the serum of these patients. There is often severe intestinal metaplasia which is commonly believed to lead to gastric carcinoma.

Chronic hypertrophic gastritis is not an inflammatory lesion of the stomach. It is a rare disorder in which the mucosal folds become prominent and covered with hyperplastic glands which secrete abundant mucus. The evidence suggests that this is a developmental abnormality (Menetrier's disease), although secondary inflammatory changes develop.

Peptic ulcers

Peptic ulcers are ulcers associated with gastric enzyme and acid-secreting mucosa. Duodenal and gastric ulcers are the commonest but they may

occur in the oesophagus, the jejunum, at a stoma (after gastroenteros-
tomy) or associated with ectopic gastric mucosa (e.g. in a Meckel's
diverticulum). On the basis of their pathology, they are divisible into
acute and chronic forms.

Acute peptic ulcers

The true incidence of these ulcers is unknown; only those which bleed or
perforate into the peritoneal cavity can be identified clinically. Since
these examples only have a short history of non-specific dyspepsia and as
acute ulcers are quite common events in the post-mortem room, their
incidence is probably quite high. Gastroscopy has revealed the presence
of many small 'haemorrhagic erosions' in some individuals, which have
been shown to heal within a few days. Acute ulcers differ from erosions in
that they are fewer in number, about 1 cm in diameter, and involve the
full thickness of the mucosa. Histologically the ulcers consist of breaches
of mucous membrane with little reaction in the underlying tissue. In the
smaller examples, the necrotic mucous membrane will be still in situ and
haemorrhage will be observed to be taking place from the capillaries of
the lamina propria.

As acute ulcers may be a consequence of operation or other
disturbance at the base of the brain and may follow severe burns,
remotely controlled humoral or nervous mechanisms are possibly the
basis of their formation.

Chronic peptic ulcers: chronic gastric ulcer and chronic duodenal ulcer

Since scars or other evidence of chronic peptic ulcer can be seen in about
10% of all autopsies, it is clear that this condition must be one of the
commonest serious disorders to affect patients. Both gastric and
duodenal ulcers are much less common in women. As with acute ulcers,
some active chronic peptic ulcers will be incidental findings in the
post-mortem room. Duodenal ulcer is at the present time about two or
three times as common as gastric ulcer, the ratio being greater in men
than in woman.

Pathology. Chronic gastric ulcers occur most commonly along the
lesser curve and the adjoining posterior wall. Duodenal ulcers are
situated in the first part, usually adjacent to the pylorus on the anterior
and posterior walls. The ulcers are usually single. When two or more
exist, they are most frequently observed in the same organ, but both
gastric and duodenal ulcers are seen in the same patient more frequently
than might be expected through chance. Apart from the fact that gastric
ulcers tend to be larger, the pathological pictures presented by the two

peptic ulcers are similar. They consist of sharply circular pits in the mucous membrane varying in size from a few millimetres to 3 or 4 cm in diameter; they are more commonly small than large. Their floors contain necrotic slough under which lies the reactive fibrous tissue typical of a chronic inflammatory process, the muscle coat having been breached. The ulcer may be shallow, or have eroded so deeply that underlying structures such as the pancreas form part of the floor.

Microscopically the ulcer floor consists of four zones. Superficially there is a purulent exudate under which is a layer of necrotic tissue. Outside the latter there is a zone of granulation tissue which merges into the outer layer of fibrous tissue. It is common to see medium-sized arteries in the ulcer floor; their lumina are usually practically occluded by endarteritis obliterans, and some in fact may contain organizing thrombi. In a proportion of cases the process of ulceration will involve the vessel wall, and, if the above regressive changes are not complete, this will lead to serious haemorrhage (haematemesis and melaena). Such eroded arteries in the ulcer floor are clearly visible to the naked eye. At the side of the ulcer, the breached muscle coat can be seen microscopically to curve upwards to meet the mucous membrane and muscularis mucosae curving downwards. The epithelium at the edge of the ulcer frequently shows atypical hyperplastic features, a reaction of epithelial cells which is common at the edge of chronic inflammatory ulcers in any situation in the body.

Progress. (1) The ulcer frequently heals. Macroscopically, the site will usually be evident because of radial ridges caused by fibrous tissue which remains under the re-epithelialized floor. Microscopically, evidence that healing has begun is shown by a reduction in the amount of granulation tissue together with a spreading in from the sides of a layer of epithelium, one cell thick. Later this becomes more complicated but specialist acid and pepsin secreting cells never return. (2) Haemorrhage may result: it may be massive through erosion of an artery in the floor, or occult as a result of seepage from the granulation tissue, in which case symptoms of chronic iron deficiency anaemia may develop. A severe haemorrhage often produces a vasovagal attack (or faint) which may pass into the condition of oligaemic (surgical) shock. (3) The ulcerative process may be so vigorous that the fibrous barrier may be inadequate and incomplete, resulting in perforation into the peritoneal cavity or erosion into neighbouring structures, e.g. pancreas. (4) Pyloric obstruction is mainly a complication of chronic duodenal ulcer but may occasionally be produced by a pre-pyloric chronic gastric ulcer. The ulcer scarring gradually narrows the lumen of the pylorus, and oedema of the mucous membrane completes the process. Proximal dilatation of the stomach results, and this may reach considerable proportions. (5) The precise relationship between gastric ulcer and carcinoma is not clear. The incidence quoted for cancer developing in a long-standing peptic ulcer (ulcer-cancer) varies from 0% to 10%, but if strict histological criteria are used, the incidence is found to be very low and nowhere near 10%. Since any gastric carcinoma is liable to ulcerate, it must be distinguished from ulcer-cancer. The criteria for the latter are (a) sharply demarcated ulcer, (b) fibrosis of the muscle coat deep to the ulcer, (c) curving up of the muscular coat at the edge of the ulcer to meet the mucosa and muscularis mucosae i.e. features of chronic peptic ulceration, (d) no carcinoma in the base of the ulcer, (e) carcinoma limited to part of the circumference of the ulcer only, (f) infiltration of the carcinoma through the muscularis mucosae. For each ulcer-cancer there are five or six ulcerated carcinomas.

Aetiology. Chronic gastric and duodenal ulcers are aetiologically quite distinct. Gastric ulcer has a greater and earlier incidence in poorer people, while the incidence of duodenal ulcer is remarkably uniform throughout the social grades of the population. This suggests that gastric ulcers may be due in part to malnutrition, an hypothesis supported by the high incidence of gastric ulcer in parts of Asia. The tendency to develop either type of ulcer is separately inherited; relatives of patients with duodenal ulcer are more than normally liable to develop duodenal ulcers but not gastric ulcers, and vice versa. Duodenal ulcers are unduly frequent in those of blood group O. Duodenal ulcers are associated with increased acid secretion whereas gastric ulcers have less acid secretion than normal. However, other factors which play a part in controlling acid secretion must also be considered, particularly neurogenic and psychosomatic stimuli. Hypothalamic stimulation is associated with peptic ulceration, whereas vagotomy reduces acid secretion. Conditions of stress, such as burns and brain injury, may lead to acute ulceration in the stomach and duodenum. Hormonal factors are also important. Adrenal corticosteroids can cause an exacerbation of a quiescent ulcer, but they are probably not able to initiate an ulcer in a subject who would otherwise remain without one. Non-insulin-secreting α-cell tumours of the pancreatic islets are sometimes associated with hypersecretion of acid and intractible peptic ulceration (Zollinger–Ellison syndrome). There is little evidence to support trauma to the gastric mucosa as being an important aetiological agent, but bile reflux may be significant.

The pathogenesis of peptic ulcers remains obscure. It is easy to see that once the breach has occurred the secretions might help to maintain the ulceration. However, both acute and chronic ulcers heal spontaneously and acute ulcers do not usually develop into chronic ones, since they do not have the anatomical localization of the latter.

Carcinoma of stomach

Deaths from malignant disease of the stomach total about 10% of all deaths from all causes of malignancy. As the prognosis is among the worst of all malignant tumours, this figure is probably representative of incidence as well as death. Only malignant disease of the bronchus and large intestine are commoner causes of death in males, and that of the breast in females. It is a disease of middle and old age with a preponderance in lower social classes. Conditions which appear to be pre-malignant are the uncommon adenomatous polyps, and gastric atrophy (see p. 140). The disease is commoner in Japan, Finland and Iceland and among people of blood group A.

Macroscopic appearances

These are variable: typically, they may appear as irregular ulcers, as fungating polypoid lesions, or as lesions which infiltrate widely in the wall but only flatten the mucosa (the so-called leather-bottle stomach or linitis plastica). When copious mucus is produced the tumour appears gelatinous and may be called a 'colloid' or 'mucoid' carcinoma. With increasing use of endoscopy, earlier recognition of carcinomas occurs and some are recognized at a superficial spreading stage, when they are confined to the mucosa or submucosa. Most carcinomas occur in the pylorus and antrum (50%) and on the lesser curve (25%), so that pyloric obstruction is a frequent complication. When the tumour occurs at the cardia (10%), it is clinically indistinguishable from a carcinoma of the lower end of the oesophagus.

Microscopic features

Most of the tumours are rather poorly differentiated adenocarcinomas. There are two basic types. In one the cells form glandular structures and secrete mucin into their lumen (so-called intestinal carcinomas). In the other (so-called diffuse carcinomas), spheroidal cells grow singly and in sheets infiltrating diffusely but without forming glands. In this type the nucleus of the cell is frequently pressed to one side by a globule of mucus in the cytoplasm (signet-ring cell). Sometimes the two patterns are mixed. The fibrous tissue stromal reaction may be well developed, especially with diffuse carcinomas, giving the leather-bottle appearance.

It is interesting that the considerable geographical variation in frequency of carcinoma is largely due to variations in the diffuse type, intestinal carcinoma being relatively constant.

Spread

Despite earlier recognition, local infiltration is usually extensive by the time the tumour is diagnosed. Infiltration through the muscularis propria is usual and microscopic spread is often far beyond the invasion assessed by the naked eye. It is of interest and probably of fundamental importance that, while spread into the oesophagus appears unimpaired, the carcinoma rarely extends into the mucosa of the duodenum.

Lymph node spread, mainly along the lesser curvature and into the porta hepatitis, is common. The left supraclavicular lymph node, adjacent to the thoracic duct, is said to be frequently involved. Blood-borne spread is very common in the liver and occurs further afield. Widespread involvement of the peritoneum occurs by transcoelomic spread and a classical finding in the female is involvement of the ovaries (Krukenberg tumours).

Pyloric stenosis

Obstruction of the stomach arises when the pylorus ceases to relax at the time when the rest of the organ undergoes peristalsis. This is most likely to occur in male infants about three weeks after birth, as a congenital defect (congenital pyloric stenosis). The pyloric muscle becomes grossly hypertrophied and there are quantitative and qualitative changes in the nerves and ganglia of Auerbach's plexus in this area. In adults, pyloric stenosis is most commonly associated with a neighbouring chronic peptic ulcer or carcinoma. The first effect of the obstruction is usually increased peristalsis which can be detected clinically. Later the stomach becomes increasingly dilated. It is not difficult to appreciate that large vomits, often projectile in nature, result from this disorder.

Carcinoma of the duodenum

Apart from chronic duodenal ulcer, gross pathological lesions in the duodenum are rare. Probably the most frequent are congenital diverticula and adenocarcinoma. When the latter develops, a likely site is the ampulla of Vater, leading to obstructive jaundice.

The jejunum and ileum

Enteritis

Eight litres of fluid reach the lumen of the intestine each 24 hours, and yet only 100 ml of this remains to be excreted in the faeces, the remainder having been absorbed, mostly in the small intestine. It is not surprising, therefore, that when diffuse lesions arise in the small bowel, there should be some imbalance between fluid accumulation and removal within the bowel lumen, resulting in diarrhoea. The most common cause of diffuse lesions in the small bowel is infection, producing gastroenteritis or enteritis, which lead to the clinical syndromes of diarrhoea and vomiting or to diarrhoea alone. In the majority of cases of gastroenteritis the cause remains unknown, either because it has not been looked for or because the agent remains bacteriologically unidentified. Salmonellae are the commonest known aetiological agents, of which there are now over 700 varieties. Other relatively common bacteria are *Staphylococcus aureus, Clostridium perfringens (welchii)*, and some strains of *Escherichia coli*. A number of enteroviruses, such as Coxsackie and Echoviruses, have also been identified. Little is known of the infective lesions in the small intestine, because so few patients die, and those that do, develop autolytic changes in the intestine with extreme rapidity. Food-poisoning is a common way by which the organisms exert their effects; the other means is by way of cross-infection. *Staphylococcus* and *Clostridium perfringens* produce food-poisoning as a result of their preformed toxins being ingested. Many cases of staphylococcal food-poisoning arise following ingestion of canned foods; *C. perfringens* infection develops in twice-cooked meats. Botulism is another rare but severe form of food-poisoning caused by the ingestion of the exotoxin of *Clostridium botulinum*. Canned meats are an important source of infection. The toxin produces widespread paralysis including the respiratory and pharyngeal muscles. *Cholera* is a severe intestinal disease due to a vibrio. It leads to massive watery diarrhoea, rapid dehydration, prostration and death due to profound shock. There is little inflammation in the intestine and the main lesion appears to be a changed permeability of the intestinal wall caused by the organism. In patients who recover, the organisms usually disappear quickly from the stools, but carrier states can occur.

Enteric fever

Enteric fever, caused by *Salmonella typhi* and *S. paratyphi* B (typhoid and paratyphoid fever), is much less frequent than it used to be, paratyphoid fever being the commoner and milder disease in Britain. Because it affects many tissues in the body and because epidemics of the disease occur from time to time, its various manifestations need to be appreciated.

Infection is almost always due to the ingestion of the pathogenic organisms in food and drink. It is particularly in uncooked food such as salads, dairy produce and ice cream that infection is likely to be transmitted. Most of the organisms are destroyed in the acid gastric juice, but if they survive they invade the lymphoid tissue of the intestine, where they multiply. After an incubation period of ten days, the clinical disease becomes evident as a septicaemia with a progressive rise in temperature, headache, epistaxis, bronchitis and abdominal symptoms of pain, constipation or diarrhoea. The lymphoid tissue of the ileum becomes swollen and after ten days of clinical disease, necrosis occurs. With separation of the slough, ulceration of the bowel occurs two or three weeks after the onset of the illness. The ulcers characteristically are longitudinal in the terminal ileum. Microscopically, the lymphoid tissue shows infiltration by large numbers of histiocytes but there is a paucity of polymorphs. The spleen is enlarged and soft and there are focal necroses in the liver with macrophage infiltration. Cardiac and striated muscle, especially the rectus abdominis muscle, shows focal necrosis (Zenker's degeneration). In the acute illness there is characteristically a leucopenia. Infection of the gall bladder is common and the resulting chronic cholecystitis may be a cause of persistent infection, with the passage of live bacteria in the faeces resulting in a 'carrier state'. These people are clinically well but are a potential danger if involved in the handling of food or water. Chronic urinary carriers may result from renal infection.

Complications of enteric fever include intestinal haemorrhage from the erosion of vessels in the ulcers, or peritonitis from perforation of these ulcers. These are most likely to occur in the third week of the clinical disease. Osteomyelitis may result from chronic infection of the medullary cavity of bones. Bronchopneumonia may complicate the initial bronchitis; there may be a peripheral neuritis.

The disease is confirmed by blood culture in the first three weeks, urine culture in the second week and stool culture after the second week. Serum agglutination tests are valuable if they show a rising titre, but people who have received typhoid antigen for protection against enteric fever may show a rising titre due to a non-specific infection—'anamnestic reaction'.

Tuberculosis

Tuberculosis of the small intestine is a disease of increasing rarity due to the decline in incidence of bovine tuberculosis. The primary infection is now rare, but still presents in Britain with lymph node enlargement in the ileocaecal region. These nodes may caseate and calcify, giving rise to tabes mesenterica, usually in the young. The primary focus in the intestine is not usually identified. In parts of Africa and Asia, primary ileocaecal tuberculosis may present with a florid proliferating granulomatous inflammatory reaction simulating malignant disease (hyperplastic ileocaecal tuberculosis). Tubercle bacilli are usually plentiful in these lesions. Secondary intestinal tuberculosis most commonly follows pulmonary infection and the swallowing of tubercle bacilli. It leads to transverse ulcers in the distal small intestine. On healing, these may cause stenosis. Infection may spread into the peritoneal cavity to give localized tuberculous peritonitis. Perforation of the intestinal ulcers usually gives a localized abscess as the infection is confined by the adhesions resulting from the preceding peritonitis.

The malabsorption syndrome

The malabsorption syndrome may be caused by lesions outside the small bowel, such as pancreatic failure or biliary tract disease, or by lesions of the small bowel itself, such as coeliac disease (idiopathic steatorrhoea, gluten-sensitive enteropathy), internal fistulae or multiple diverticula in the small intestine. In coeliac disease the presence of gluten in the diet results in a chronic inflammatory process in the mucosa of the small intestine. The normal villous architecture is lost; the villi become shorter and broader and the crypts longer. The mucosa has an increased number of lymphoid cells in it and malabsorption results. A gluten-free diet returns the mucosa to normal. A genetic predisposition to this condition exists, for HLA-B8 occurs in approximately 80% of patients (its occurrence in the normal population in the UK being about 25%).

Similar changes in the mucosa may be seen in tropical sprue but they do not respond to gluten withdrawal. The probable cause is an unidentified infection.

Infection of the lumen of the small bowel with a flagellate protozoon, *Giardia lamblia*, also causes malabsorption without usually much morphological abnormality in the mucosa. The parasite is best identified in jejunal aspiration.

Crohn's disease

This inflammatory process of obscure origin appears to be becoming more frequent. Its commonly used synonym, regional ileitis, indicates that the ileum is usually implicated. However, it is now appreciated that it may involve any part of the gastrointestinal tract, although the ileum is the commonest site of involvement. Most cases present in the third decade, although it may occur at any age. Both men and women are affected. The inflammatory process produces 'skip lesion', i.e. inflamed portions of bowel in between normal ones. The affected bowel is thickened and firm. There are serosal adhesions and frequently fistulae between one loop of bowel and another or to the skin or bladder. Anal fistulae and perianal ulceration are common. The mucosa shows ulceration with oedematous surviving mucosa giving a cobblestone appearance. Histologically, the dominant features are submucous oedema with dilated lymphatics, chronic inflammatory foci extending through the thickness of the bowel wall, some of the foci being lymphoid follicles and others granulomata containing epithelioid cells and Langhans giant cells, but never caseation. The bowel lumen is narrowed, the mucous membrane ulcerated and fissures run deep into the bowel wall or form fistulae with neighbouring structures. The serosal surface shows chronic inflammation and oedema. Regional lymphadenopathy is associated with giant cell granulomas in the lymph nodes.

The narrowed segment of bowel is liable to produce intestinal obstruction. The ulcerated mucosa results in blood loss and iron deficiency anaemia, and the diseased terminal ileum leads to megaloblastic anaemia due to malabsorption of vitamin B_{12}. The disease is progressive, for although it is amenable to surgery, recurrences are common.

Small intestine obstruction

Obstruction of the *small intestine*, because of its length, its mesenteric attachment, and free movement, most frequently results from a band of connective tissue lying across it as in strangulated hernias, or because it gets twisted (volvulus). In both instances the blood supply is cut off and infarction occurs. Intestinal obstruction may be a complication of prolonged operative handling or of infection originating elsewhere in the peritoneal cavity, because of the development of the state of paralytic ileus. In newborn infants it may be due to inspissated meconium associated with the condition of mucoviscidosis (see p. 174). In older children it may be due to intussusception where one portion of bowel passes into another, dragging its mesentery with it and resulting in obstruction to the blood supply and infarction of the bowel. The commonest site is the terminal ileum (intussusceptum) which passes into the colon (intussuscipiens). In children this may be due to adenovirus infection producing hyperplasia of lymphoid tissue which gets carried along the bowel lumen by peristalsis. In the large intestine, carcinoma is the commonest cause of intussusception. Inflammatory diseases such as tuberculosis or Crohn's disease may produce a stricture. Foreign bodies in the lumen may also cause obstruction. The first effect of obstruction of the small bowel is increased peristaltic activity of the viable bowel proximal to the obstruction, often detected clinically because of the increased intensity of the bowel sounds. Later the bowel will dilate, when the bowel sounds will become reduced. When peristalsis ceases in the dilated bowel, this segment now becomes a source of obstruction to the alimentary canal higher up, and this is what occurs in paralytic ileus. Small-bowel obstruction is a highly dangerous state and will lead to death unless relieved. This is because the obstructed bowel is very liable to infection from the bacteria within the lumen and general peritonitis will ensue.

Meckel's diverticulum

This congenital abnormality is found in 2% of the population. It occurs at a distance of about 0.6 m from the ileocaecal valve as a true diverticulum, i.e. lined by mucous membrane and covered by muscle. It may be connected to the umbilicus by a fibrous band, in which remnants of the vitellointestinal duct may persist as a vitelline cyst. The diverticulum may produce symptoms because of the peptic ulceration which is liable to develop in the ectopic gastric mucous membrane commonly present.

Neoplasms

Neoplasms of the small intestine are rare and include argentaffinoma (carcinoid tumour), leiomyoma and leiomyosarcoma and malignant lymphoma. Apart from those in the ampulla of Vater, carcinomas are rare. Polyps may be found in the Peutz–Jeghers syndrome, which are tumour-like malformations rather than true neoplasms. Argentaffinomas arise from the cells of the diffuse endocrine system of the gut. The tumours are yellow and consist of nests of orderly cells infiltrating through the muscle coat of the bowel. The tumour may metastasize to regional lymph nodes and liver. When it does so it may give the 'malignant carcinoid' syndrome associated with the overproduction of 5-hydroxytryptamine (5-HT) and kinins. This syndrome consists of attacks of skin flushing, diarrhoea and pulmonary stenosis due to endocardial fibrosis of the right side of the heart. The syndrome does not occur without hepatic metastases.

The appendix

Acute appendicitis

This common acute abdominal emergency carried a considerable mortality in the pre-antibiotic era as a result of the liability to general peritonitis following perforation of the inflamed organ. However, the disease is now much less serious as the peritonitis responds to available antibiotic therapy.

Macroscopic picture

The affected part of the organ is usually oedematous and blotchy red with a fibrinous or fibrinopurulent exudate on the surface. In the more advanced cases, the wall becomes necrotic or gangrenous. Frequently the inflammation is confined to the distal half which is then sharply demarcated from the more normal proximal end. When this happens, a hardened pellet of faeces, a 'faecolith', may be seen filling the lumen of the inflamed section. The mucous membrane is ulcerated and the lumen may contain pus. In a proportion of cases, especially when gangrene supervenes, perforation of the wall occurs, with the result that the inflammation extends to the surrounding tissues and, in some cases, to the whole of the peritoneal cavity. The contents of the peritoneal cavity have a great ability to localize infections and, as a result, an 'appendix abscess' is a frequent end-result of perforation.

Microscopic picture

Many inflamed appendices producing symptoms may look nearly normal macroscopically, but show evidence of infection histologically. The whole wall of the affected part shows the classical features of acute inflammation including the formation of an exudate on the surface. In gangrenous appendicitis the inflammatory exudate brings about obstruction to the blood supply so that part of the wall becomes necrotic. In the more rarely observed early cases, the inflammation will be limited to an ulcerated area of the mucous membrane and the tissues immediately beneath.

Progress

It is not known whether acute appendicitis can regress without antibiotics, though this is probable. Once diagnosed, surgical removal is the rule. The only certain occasion when the acute inflammation becomes chronic is after a perforation which subsequently becomes localized.

Aetiology

The appendix is a blind-ended tube whose lumen contains bacteria. It is not surprising, therefore, that once the mucous membrane has become ulcerated the wall should become infected. A wide variety of faecal organisms are isolated from inflamed appendices. A large number of inflamed appendices contain faecoliths and when these are present the inflammation and destruction of tissue are usually maximal at the site of the faecolith. It is probable that muscular constriction in this area leads to an initial ischaemic necrosis of the mucosa with subsequent inflammation. In the many cases without faecoliths, a possible explanation is that muscle spasm or submucosal lymphoid hyperplasia at the proximal end interferes with effective drainage of the distal portion; distension then occurs leading to ischaemia of the mucosa and infection from the bowel lumen. The prevalence of acute appendicitis is greatest in people with a Western diet, but the precise causal relationship is still to be elucidated.

Following obstruction to the lumen of the appendix, the inflammation may resolve to leave a mucocoele. Rarely, this lining epithelium becomes neoplastic to form a cystadenoma or cystadenocarcinoma of the appendix. Rupture of these lesions into the peritoneal cavity may result in pseudomyxoma peritonei (see p. 197).

Neoplasms

Argentaffinoma or carcinoid tumour of the appendix consists of a small yellow nodule, usually at the distal end, and is most commonly picked up as an incidental finding in routine appendicectomy specimens. Those at the distal end rarely give further trouble, but those at the proximal end are more likely to metastasize and give rise to the carcinoid syndrome (p. 111).

The large intestine

The faeces are more fluid in the caecum than the rectum, because water is absorbed to some extent in the large bowel. Mucus secretion is more active in this section of the intestine than higher up and becomes excessive under conditions of diffuse stimulation, such as in infection by dysentery organisms, in ulcerative colitis, or in cases of nervous irritability (mucous colitis).

Dysentery

Members of the genus *Shigella* are responsible for *bacillary dysentery*, of which *S. sonnei* is outstandingly the most common in Britain, the next most frequent being the organism of Flexner dysentery. Sonne dysentery is also the mildest form, producing usually only diarrhoea. The more severe variants result in the passage of increased amounts of blood and mucus. Macroscopically, the large bowel is congested and, in the severe cases, is covered with many shallow ulcers containing purulent exudate and affecting particularly the tips of the mucosal folds. Microscopically, the mucous membrane is infiltrated with inflammatory cells, polymorphs predominating in the acute cases and lymphocytes and plasma cells in the more chronic cases.

Amoebic dysentery has been described earlier (see p. 38).

Diverticulosis and diverticulitis

Diverticula, consisting of herniations of mucous membrane and submucosa through the muscularis (i.e. 'false' diverticula in contrast to 'true' diverticula which are pouches covered by all layers of the bowel wall and which are congenital in origin), are common in the colon in populations with a Western diet, increasing in frequency with age, being uncommon under 35. They are usually multiple and most frequently located in the sigmoid colon where they form small outpushings which may extend into the appendices epiploicae between the mesenteric and antimesenteric taeniae. Excessive bowel contraction is considered to be an important factor in making them become larger. The muscle coat of the bowel in the affected area is grossly thickened and firm. Circular muscle fibres cause indentation of the bowel lumen. Diverticulosis is the name given to the presence of multiple diverticula, when present in the symptomless state. The mucous membrane of the diverticula is, however, liable to ulcerate, and the surrounding serous coat then becomes the seat of episodes of inflammation (or diverticulitis) which may lead to abdominal pain. On occasions, the ulceration is followed by stricture formation or by perforation into the peritoneal cavity. Bleeding is another important complication.

Chronic ulcerative colitis

This is a distressing disease affecting any age group but presenting most commonly in early adult life. It is of obscure aetiology, and leads to the passage of a large number of stools in the day usually containing blood and mucus. Spontaneous regression can take place, but the disease is liable to become chronic, and to require extensive surgical excision for the amelioration of the symptoms.

Macroscopic picture

The disease may affect any part or all of the large bowel but it is usually most severe in the descending colon and rectum. Many cases appear to start in the rectum as idiopathic proctitis. In the affected areas, the whole mucosa is diseased, differing from Crohn's disease where islands of normal mucosa are interspersed in diseased areas to produce 'skip lesions'. The inflammation usually stops short at the ileocaecal valve, but where this is incompetent there may be a 'backwash ileitis'. The affected bowel is shortened and the wall thickened with loss of normal haustrations. The mucosa is congested and covered by shallow ulcers. These rarely extend into the muscle coat and inflammation is confined to the superficial layers, unlike the transmural inflammation and deep fissures of Crohn's disease. In severe cases, the neighbouring ulcers may coalesce leaving tags of surviving mucous membrane to project from the ulcerated surface. These tags may be numerous and at times show reactive proliferation, so that the bowel appears to be covered with polyps (pseudo-polyposis coli), similar to the rare hereditary condition, polyposis coli. Despite the extensive inflammation and ulceration, reactive fibrosis of the underlying wall is rare. Occasionally, fulminating cases occur in which the colon becomes grossly dilated and friable. This state of toxic megacolon carries a high mortality, and surgery is difficult because of the friability of the bowel. It is in this state that perforation of the colon is most likely in ulcerative colitis. Other complications include iron deficiency anaemia, hypoproteinaemia, arthritis, skin lesions of pyoderma gangrenosum and erythema nodosum, and lastly carcinoma of the colon. Carcinoma is liable to develop in cases of long-standing ulcerative colitis, although the mucosa is usually atrophic at this time. The presence of carcinoma in the colon can often be predicted by the presence of glandular atypia on rectal biopsy. It is a wise precaution to keep long-standing cases under review for this reason.

Microscopic picture

Though it is called 'ulcerative colitis', actual ulceration is only seen in the more severe cases. It is essentially a disease of the mucosa. There are increased numbers of lymphocytes and plasma cells in the lamina propria and often polymorphonuclear leucocytes in the gland tubules ('crypt abscesses'). The epithelial cells are depleted of mucus and in chronic cases there is distortion of the gland architecture. Only in toxic dilatation is there significant inflammation in the submucosa and muscularis propria.

Crohn's disease

This disease affects the large bowel and may be difficult to distinguish from ulcerative colitis (see p. 152) but the rectum is often spared.

Pseudomembranous colitis

This condition derives its unsatisfactory name from the fact that there is an exudate (the pseudomembrane) lying on top of and adherent to the mucous membrane. It starts as focal lesions but, if it progresses, these become confluent and the whole of the wall may become necrotic.

The disease was first described in the 19th century; most cases seen nowadays occur in people who have taken antibiotics. It usually presents as diarrhoea. Sigmoidoscopy reveals small yellowish flecks on the mucosa, which later enlarge to form plaques. Some cases are mild and self-limiting, but in others (particularly elderly debilitated patients) it can result in death. The cause is thought to be a toxin-producing *Clostridium difficile* which may grow as a result of the alteration in bowel flora produced by antibiotics. Occasional cases occur without preceding antibiotic therapy.

Ischaemic colitis

This is an uncommon condition which is seen particularly at the splenic flexure in elderly people. This is the area of the colon with the poorest blood supply, being at the margin of supply of the superior and inferior mesenteric artery. It is therefore vulnerable to a sudden drop in blood pressure or other vascular disturbances. The changes produced vary depending on the severity and duration of the reduction in blood supply. If it is severe and prolonged, then infarction of the whole thickness of the bowel occurs. If it is mild and transient, then death of the superficial part of the mucosa occurs followed by regeneration. Between these extremes there are some cases where the initial damage affects the mucosa and submucosa but, during the healing phase, fibrosis occurs resulting in narrowing of the bowel which gives rise to obstruction.

Polyps

The word 'polyp' is used to describe almost any lump protruding from an epithelial surface. The commonest polyps in the large bowel are neoplastic, but there are also hamartomatous and inflammatory polyps, and a miscellaneous group.

Neoplastic polyps are the most important. They arise from the columnar epithelium and have two growth patterns. The common variety is a tubular adenoma which is a rounded lump on a narrow stalk, having a tubular gland pattern. They are often multiple and are most common in the sigmoid colon and rectum. The villous adenoma typically occurs in the rectum, is usually solitary and consists of finger-like outgrowths of epithelium. It is probably best to think of these two as ends of a spectrum rather than distinct lesions, for mixtures of growth patterns are seen and the abnormal epithelial cells in each type all show a degree of dysplasia. While the abnormal growth is confined to the mucosa, the polyps are regarded as benign (or, more accurately, pre-malignant), but as soon as the cells breach the muscularis mucosae their behaviour alters to that of a carcinoma. The larger the polyp, the more likely is invasion. These polyps become increasingly common in the middle-aged and elderly in populations with a Western diet. In familial polyposis coli (inherited as a Mendelian dominant), multiple neoplastic polyps develop in early adult life. If the colon is not removed, the development of carcinoma is certain.

Hamartomas are tumour-like malformations. Juvenile polyps consist of cystic glands and loose connective tissue. They cause symptoms usually because of bleeding. Peutz–Jeghers polyps consist of glands, connective tissue and muscle; the polyps often occur elsewhere in the gastrointestinal gland and are associated with mucosal pigmentation in the Peutz–Jeghers syndrome. They cause symptoms because of bleeding and sometimes because of obstruction. These polyps are not regarded as pre-malignant.

Inflammatory polyps occur in chronic inflammatory bowel disease. There are two types: one consists of inflammatory granulation tissue arranged in the form of a polyp; the other, sometimes called a pseudopolyp, occurs when intact mucosa becomes surrounded and undermined by an ulcerating area—the resulting island appearing polypoid.

The commonest member of the miscellaneous group is the metaplastic polyp. Metaplastic polyps are small (2–3 mm diameter) sessile lesions which are asymptomatic and are composed of slightly papillary epithelium which was originally thought to resemble small intestinal mucosa. They are thought to be benign.

Malignant tumours

The most important malignant tumour of the · large intestine is carcinoma. This is one of the commonest forms of malignancy in Western countries, being comparable with carcinoma of the lung. However, since approximately 50% of carcinomas of the large intestine are cured by surgery, the death rate for colonic and rectal carcinoma is less than that for lung cancer. The tumour is most common in older people, rectal carcinoma being about twice as common in men as in women. Colonic carcinoma is more common in women. Most of the tumours are within range of the sigmoidoscope, about half occurring in the rectum and a quarter in the sigmoid colon. Caecum and ascending colon are important but less common sites for carcinoma. Tumours of the rectum usually carry a better prognosis than those of the caecum and ascending colon because they present earlier. This is because the distal tumours frequently cause obstruction of the solid faeces, but obstruction of liquid faeces in the caecum is late. The tumour in the caecum may present as chronic iron deficiency anaemia from intestinal blood loss or it may present with an abdominal mass and right iliac fossa pain. On the left side of the large bowel, alteration of bowel habit and the passage of bright red blood per rectum are more likely presenting symptoms. Predisposing factors include neoplastic polyps and ulcerative colitis.

Macroscopic picture

The carcinomas usually take one of three forms: polypoid tumours, ulcers with slightly raised edges, or stenosing (annular) tumours. Ulcerating tumours are much the commonest form for rectal carcinomas, whereas polypoid forms are the most frequent in the ascending colon. Stenosing tumours occur more often in the colon than the rectum. In the later stages the carcinoma completely encircles the bowel wall. Stenosing carcinomas of the colon can give rise to large-bowel obstruction, the muscular wall of the bowel above becoming hypertrophied and then dilated. Such obstructed patients are not as acutely ill as those who have small bowel obstruction.

Microscopic picture

Almost all the carcinomas are gland-forming adenocarcinomas of varying degrees of differentiation, some being anaplastic. Occasional tumours are of 'signet-ring' pattern.

Spread

This is often limited to the bowel wall at the time of diagnosis. Spread may be by direct infiltration which, in the case of the rectum, can extend into neighbouring structures such as the bladder. Extension to the peritoneal coat may lead to ascites or perforation with subsequent peritonitis. Lymphatic spread occurs first to regional lymph nodes. Blood-borne spread tends to occur late, usually to the liver first. A careful study has shown that the five-year survival bears a direct relation to the extent of spread at the time of operation. In Dukes' classification Stage A, the tumour is confined to the bowel wall; in Stage B, it has spread directly through the bowel wall; in Stage C, there is lymph node involvement. The corrected five-year survivals for these three stages are 98%, 78% and 30%, respectively.

Other malignant neoplasms of the large intestine are rare but they include lymphomas, carcinoid tumours and leiomyosarcomas.

Carcinoma of the anus and anal canal

Carcinoma of the rectum is about 30 times as common as carcinoma of the anus. The tumours of the latter are usually typical squamous cell carcinomas, although occasionally poorly differentiated carcinomas may mimic basal cell carcinomas. These *basaloid* carcinomas should not be confused with true basal cell carcinomas that may arise in the hair-bearing skin of the anus. Squamous cell and basaloid carcinomas may spread by lymphatics, both in the direction of the inferior mesenteric vein branches and to the inguinal group of lymph nodes. Malignant melanoma also occurs at this site.

Hirschsprung's disease

This is due to a congenital defect in the ganglion cells of Meissner's and Auerbach's plexus, usually in the rectosigmoid junction, and resulting in a failure of peristalsis in this area. The affected bowel is contracted but the large bowel proximal to the obstruction becomes massively dilated and requires surgical resection of the affected aganglionic segment. In adults, an idiopathic form of megacolon is seen, but here ganglion cells in the bowel wall appear normal.

Haemorrhoids (piles)

These are dilated submucosal venous channels which lie immediately below the mucous membrane in the anal canal. They are extremely common in the older age groups and are liable to give rise to recurrent slight haemorrhage, especially after defecation. Pain and prolapse also occur. The cause in most cases is obscure but the erect posture adopted by human beings and straining at defecation are important factors in their genesis. The recent development of haemorrhoids in a middle-aged or elderly patient should always arouse the suspicion of a carcinoma in the rectum.

Anal fissure

Anal fissure is a longitudinal ulcer in the anus, usually in the midline posteriorly and below the level of the pectinate line. It probably results from the damage caused by passing hard faeces.

Fistula-in-ano

This is an inflammatory condition in which a track links the columnar lined mucosa near the pectinate line to another point, usually in the perianal skin, though sometimes it opens in the rectum. The commonest cause is infection of the anal glands. It may occur on its own, though it is sometimes associated with other conditions such as Crohn's disease.

Specific anal infections

The rectum and anus may be affected by venereal infections such as gonorrhoea, syphilis, condylomata acuminata and lymphogranuloma inguinale. The inflammatory changes are similar to those seen when the infection occurs on the genitalia.

17

The Alimentary System (II)

The liver

The liver receives, by way of the portal vein, the blood which has drained the gastrointestinal tract, pancreas and spleen, and, after admixture with that in the hepatic artery, the blood passes via the sinusoids in the lobules to the central veins and then, via the hepatic vein, almost immediately into the right atrium of the heart. It is not surprising, therefore, that the organ should frequently show degenerative changes arising as a consequence of disturbances of nutrition and circulation. Cloudy swelling, fatty change, atrophy, necrosis, fibrosis, chronic venous congestion, amyloid disease are all reactions which take place in this organ. Some have already been described in the section on general pathology, and some will come to light in the description of the specific hepatic lesions in this chapter. The liver is an organ which is capable of considerable regeneration of its parenchyma following necrosis of the component cells due to various agents. The liver is also an important component of the reticuloendothelial system by virtue of the Kupffer cells lining the sinus walls and others in the portal tracts. It takes part, therefore, in the many activities of the system; for example, haemosiderin is stored in the Kupffer cells when the supply of body iron for haemopoiesis exceeds the demand. Finally, the liver participates in haemopoiesis in the fetus, and this ability may be observed in postnatal life under abnormal conditions, such as in haemolytic disease of the newborn, and neoplastic diseases of the bone marrow.

In discussing the pathology of the liver we shall refer to the concept of the classic hepatic lobule which is described as a polygon with a central vein and with portal tracts at the corners, blood flowing from portal tracts via sinusoids to the central vein. In the portal tracts there are branches of the hepatic artery, the portal vein and tributaries of the bile ducts. The parenchymal cells at the junction of the portal tract and lobule form the limiting plate. A complementary view of liver structure is to think of the parenchyma as being constructed of secretory units (or acini) producing bile which flows to bile ducts.

Infections of the liver

Viral hepatitis
Many viruses affect the liver but this term is usually taken to imply

hepatitis caused by hepatitis A virus (HA), hepatitis B virus (HB) and an ill-defined group called non-A and non-B. Other viral infections include yellow fever, cytomegalovirus, rubella and infectious mononucleosis.

Hepatitis A is the classical infectious hepatitis with a short incubation period (two to six weeks) occurring in epidemics or sporadic cases and spread chiefly by the faecal–oral route. It presents with jaundice and may be a mild or severe disease, depending on the host response to the virus, but it is seldom fatal. On microscopy, the affected liver shows focal necrosis of parenchymal cells, predominantly centrilobular, associated with lymphocytes. There is also inflammation in the portal tracts. In severe cases, this necrosis is massive and at post-mortem the liver has a yellow wrinkled appearance called 'acute yellow atrophy'. Usually recovery occurs, the virus is eliminated and chronic liver disease does not develop.

Hepatitis B was discovered to be the cause of serum hepatitis, which has a long incubation period (six weeks to six months) and follows transfusion or injection with infected material. The antigen was originally found in an Australian aborigine, and subsequent work has shown a spectrum of disease which is wider than the original idea of serum hepatitis. The host response is crucial in the way the disease gives rise to symptoms. Following infection, the virus may be completely eliminated without any sign of disease. Alternatively, there may be quite a vigorous reaction and an acute hepatitis occurs with histology similar to that of hepatitis A; this may produce massive necrosis but recovery usually occurs. Some patients (whether or not they have had an acute illness) become chronic carriers and some of these develop cirrhosis. The reasons for the variability in the manifestations of infection are not known. In general, infection with hepatitis B virus is more severe with a worse prognosis than hepatitis A. Hepatitis nonA-nonB is now the commonest form of hepatitis transmitted by blood transfusion and is similar in prognosis to hepatitis B.

Other infections

These do not occur very frequently in Britain. Infection may spread to the liver by way of the portal vein from fulminating acute inflammation in the abdominal cavity, such as suppurative appendicitis giving rise to *pyaemic abscesses*. Infection may also spread by way of the hepatic artery to the liver in cases of systemic infections, especially bacterial endocarditis. Acute inflammation of the intrahepatic bile ducts (acute cholangitis) may give abscesses in portal tracts (suppurative cholangitis). This is usually secondary to obstruction of large bile ducts by stones or tumour in the common bile duct or tumour in the head of the pancreas. *Amoebic abscesses* occur most commonly in the right lobe of the liver. They have a ragged necrotic lining containing amoebae. Most of the necrosis is produced by cytolytic enzymes of the amoebae and inflammation is usually slight. The necrotic contents of the abscess are reddish-brown, resembling anchovy sauce. *Actinomycotic abscesses* are usually secondary to infection in the region of the appendix. Multiple abscesses produce a honeycomb pattern in the liver. The lesions contain colonies of *Actinomyces israeli* surrounded by histiocytes and poly-morphs. These colonies produce the characteristic sulphur granules seen in actinomycosis. *Weil's disease* is due to infection with the spirochaete *Leptospira icterohaemorrhagica*. It is transmitted in the urine of infected rats and passes through the skin during immersion in infected water. It causes swelling of liver cells and bile stasis. Necrosis is usually slight and focal. There is also involvement of kidneys (interstitial nephritis and tubular necrosis), heart and skeletal muscle. Granulomatous inflamma-tion may be due to tuberculosis, sarcoidosis, syphilis or liver flukes. Hyatid cysts, the cystic stage of infection by *Taenia echinococcus*, have been described earlier (see p. 41).

Chronic hepatitis

Though some of the infections mentioned above are 'chronic hepatitis' in the widest sense, the term is used in a more restricted fashion nowadays. Chronic hepatitis is clinically defined as an inflammation in the liver associated with abnormal liver function tests continuing without improvement for three months or more. There are several patterns of associated pathology seen in the liver. *Chronic persistent hepatitis* (CPH) shows chronic inflammatory cells in the portal tracts but no other abnormality. *Chronic lobular hepatitis* (CLH) shows death of parenchy-mal cells focally, associated with lymphocytes. *Chronic active (aggressive) hepatitis* (CAH) shows inflammatory cells in the portal tracts with death of some cells in the limiting plate area ('piecemeal necrosis') and disturbance of the lobular architecture. These patterns of inflammation are not distinct diseases, but they are indicators of prognosis: CPH and CLH seldom progress to cirrhosis and tend to remit, whereas CAH often progresses to cirrhosis. The aetiological agents involved in causing chronic hepatitis include most of those associated with cirrhosis.

Necrosis of the liver

Liver necrosis, apart from that associated with the infections already described, may be focal or zonal. Focal necroses are found at random throughout the liver and are a feature of typhoid fever and of diphtheria. Zonal necroses occur in relation to the liver lobule. Yellow fever produces midzonal necrosis associated with the formation of eosinophi-lic, hyaline, dead liver cells (*Councilman bodies*). Centrilobular necrosis is a feature of anoxic states, such as chronic venous congestion, or of toxic states, such as carbon tetrachloride poisoning. Periportal necrosis is found in eclampsia of pregnancy and in phosphorous poisoning.

Drug-induced liver disease

The liver is a major site of metabolism of many substances ingested into the body. It is not surprising, therefore, that some of these substances cause damage to the organ. Fatty change and focal necrosis are frequent results of toxic substances, but chronic active hepatitis, cirrhosis, granulomatous hepatitis, vascular abnormalities and benign and malignant tumours can all be induced by chemicals.

Drug-induced jaundice is a clinical problem and a drug history must always be sought in a jaundiced patient. Some drugs predictably produce jaundice if given in large enough doses, others only occasionally produce disease and then in an unpredictable fashion. The resulting jaundice may be predominantly due to retention of bile within the liver (cholestatic effect), or to death of cells with an inflammatory reaction (hepatitic effect). Mixed pictures may be seen. Table 5 gives some examples of drugs causing jaundice.

Table 5. Examples of some drugs causing jaundice.

	Hepatitic/necrotic	*Cholestatic*
Predictable	Chloroform	Anabolic steroids
Unpredictable	Halothane	Chlorpromazine

Alcohol-induced liver disease

The commonest cause of liver damage in Britian is alcohol. Heavy drinkers almost always show fatty change in parenchymal cells; this change is predictable, dose related and reversible. Some drinkers develop a hepatitis which is characterized by dead liver cells, a neutrophil infiltrate in the lobules, and a curious degenerative change (known as Mallory's hyaline) in the cytoplasm of some parenchymal cells. The hyaline change and the dead cells tend to occur in the centrilobular areas. Centrilobular sclerosis occurs when connective tissue is laid down around the central veins, sometimes obliterating them. Cirrhosis develops in at least 20% of chronic alcoholics, dose and duration of abuse being important determinants. The factors which determine whether an alcoholic develops cirrhosis are not fully understood, but it seems likely that the fibrosis and nodular regeneration of the cirrhosis are related to the cell necrosis of hepatitis, rather than to simple fatty change.

Cirrhosis

Though originally applied to the tawny colour of some diseased livers, the word 'cirrhosis' is now used to refer to a group of chronic liver diseases characterized by fibrosis and nodular regeneration occurring as a result of liver cell necrosis. The liver has a good capacity for regeneration and after one sublethal insult may restore itself to normal. However, in chronic damage, where liver cells are being killed at the same time as repair processes are proceeding, disordered parenchymal cell regeneration occurs and nodules develop. These regeneration nodules lack central veins and other normal connections and are functionally inefficient. With the associated fibrosis, they produce the main clinical effects of cirrhosis, namely portal hypertension and functional failure.

Classification

No entirely satisfactory classification is available but cirrhosis may be characterized in terms of aetiology or morphology.

Aetiology

The cause of many cases of cirrhosis is not known and these are called cryptogenic. Excess alcohol is the commonest aetiological agent in Britain. Other factors include hepatitis B virus, prolonged cholestasis, immunological disease (such as primary biliary cirrhosis), metabolic disorders (haemochromatosis, Wilson's disease, α_1-antitrypsin deficiency) and, very rarely, prolonged severe cardiac failure.

Morphology

Early attempts at understanding cirrhosis involved post-mortem observation of the appearance of the liver and gave rise to the classification of cirrhosis as portal (Laennec's or fine), post-necrotic (coarse), and biliary (obstructive and Hanot's). This classification has not proved satisfactory. Nowadays, the morphological types referred to are: (1) *micronodular*, where every lobule is destroyed and the nodules are relatively uniform, measuring less than 4 mm in diameter, and (2) *macronodular*, where some lobules may be spared, the nodules are irregular in size and some measure more than 4 mm in diameter. A complication in this simple scheme is that large nodules may develop in the 'end-stage liver' no matter what the original pattern. Alcoholic cirrhosis is micronodular in its development, whereas hepatitis B and other agents associated with a chronic active hepatitis more often produce a macronodular cirrhosis. Biopsy of a macronodular liver may not be diagnostic of cirrhosis, for normal lobules may be present and regeneration nodules may not be included in the specimen.

Macroscopic appearances

The liver in micronodular cirrhosis may be small or it may be large and fatty. In macronodular cirrhosis it is usually small and coarsely scarred.

On section, the regeneration nodules are seen as masses of pale liver tissue separated by fibrous strands. The liver of biliary cirrhosis is green due to cholestasis and the nodularity is very fine. If there is large-duct obstruction, the cut surface of the liver may show dilated bile ducts and the cause of the obstruction such as gall-stone, stricture of the common bile duct, carcinoma of the bile duct or head of pancreas, or congenital atresia may be apparent. In haemochromatosis, the liver is stained mahogany brown by haemosiderin, and in cardiac cirrhosis there is evidence of long-standing passive venous congestion.

Microscopic appearances

The microscopic features of cirrhosis are destruction of the normal architecture, extensive fibrosis, and the presence of regeneration nodules (which lack central veins). The degree of activity of the disease process causing the cirrhosis can be assessed from the amount of inflammation and liver cell destruction. The cause of the cirrhosis can often be identified from the histological appearances.

Alcoholic cirrhosis is micronodular and usually shows fatty change. Sometimes the features of alcoholic hepatitis are superimposed on the cirrhosis. With hepatitis B virus disease, the viral particles can be identified in the parenchymal cells.

Biliary cirrhosis may be primary or secondary. Primary biliary (Hanot's) cirrhosis occurs in middle-aged women and is believed to be an autoimmune disease: antimitochondrial antibodies are demonstrated in the serum. A non-suppurative pericholangitis occurs, destroying bile ducts. Giant cell granulomas may be present. Bile stasis is apparent in canaliculi and parenchymal cells. Portal tracts become expanded and contain abnormal ductules. There is gradual destruction of liver tissue but regeneration nodules of fully established cirrhosis are rare. These patients show clinical evidence of long-standing biliary obstruction with cutaneous xanthomata.

In *secondary biliary cirrhosis*, the features of bile duct obstruction (see p. 166) are apparent. The severity of bile stasis is such that liver cells die leaving pools of necrotic bile-stained debris (bile necroses or bile lakes). There is gradual destruction of parenchyma but regeneration nodules of fully established cirrhosis are rare.

Haemochromatosis is due to abnormal intestinal absorption of iron. It is rare in women during their reproductive life because they lose iron in menstruation. There is massive deposition of iron in liver parenchymal cells, Kupffer cells lining sinusoids and in portal tracts. This leads to progressive fibrosis and cirrhosis. Other organs involved include the pancreas, heart, gonads and skin. Skin pigmentation is due partly to iron deposition around skin appendages and partly to increased melanin. This pigmentation together with diabetes from pancreatic destruction have given the alternative name of 'bronzed diabetes' for this disease.

Iron overload from other causes (such as overtransfusion) used to be called haemosiderosis and was not thought to cause cirrhosis. It seems more likely, however, that cirrhosis is related to the degree of overload and will develop if enough iron accumulates, whatever the cause.

Wilson's disease (*hepatolenticular degeneration*) is caused by copper deposition in liver, brain and kidney due to failure of biliary copper excretion; serum caeruloplasmin levels are usually low. This results in cirrhosis, degeneration of basal ganglia in the brain, aminoaciduria and staining of the cornea (Kayser–Fleischer ring).

α_1-*antitrypsin deficiency* is a rare metabolic disorder in which α_1-antitrypsin is not released from hepatic parenchymal cells, where it is manufactured. The deficiency in the plasma leads to pulmonary emphysema and the abnormality in the liver is associated with cirrhosis.

Cardiac cirrhosis is an uncommon consequence of long-standing passive venous congestion of the liver, usually due to rheumatic or congenital heart disease. Liver damage is maximal in the centre of lobules, resulting in fibrosis in this area and link-up of one central area with another (paradoxical lobulation). Regeneration nodules of surviving liver cells results in a fine cirrhosis.

Complications

These fall into three main categories: (1) portal hypertension, (2) liver cell failure, and (3) tumour. Because of obstruction to the blood supply through the liver, pressure rises in the portal vein and causes dilatation of anastomotic veins in the lower end of the oesophagus (oesophageal varices) and in the anterior abdominal wall (caput Medusae). Rupture of oesophageal varices results in massive heamorrhage into the gastrointestinal tract and is one of the major causes of death. Portal hypertension also causes splenomegaly and the enlarged spleen shows evidence of congestion and old haemorrhage, resulting in brown fibrous nodules (Gamna–Gandy bodies). Splenomegaly may cause a depression of all the cellular elements in the peripheral blood (hypersplenism). Liver cell failure may manifest itself in many ways. There may be mental deterioration leading to coma due to failure to detoxify ammonia. Failure to inactivate oestrogens may cause gynaecomastia, testicular atrophy, spider naevi in the skin and 'liver palms'. Failure to synthesize albumin may result in hypoproteinaemia and oedema. Hypoproteinaemia is probably also a contributory factor in producing the ascites of cirrhosis, although portal hypertension and fluid retention (secondary aldosteronism) play their part (see p. 211). Failure to synthesize clotting factors, notably prothrombin and Factor VII, results in coagulation disorders. This may be accentuated by increased fibrinolytic activity of blood which is found in many cirrhotic patients. Cirrhosis is a very common finding in patients with primary carcinoma of the liver. In Britain about 15% of patients dying with cirrhosis have a primary liver cell carcinoma. The cirrhosis is usually macronodular in type.

Extrahepatic obstruction

It has already been indicated that jaundice may develop as a result of intrahepatic disease, such as infective hepatitis and in some cases of cirrhosis. It also arises in those relatively uncommon cases of haemolytic anaemia when the bilirubin formed from the excessive breakdown of red cells cannot be cleared by the liver effectively. The third way in which jaundice occurs is because an obstruction develops in a large bile duct often outside the liver (extrahepatic obstruction). This may arise because (1) carcinoma of the head of the pancreas obstructs the common bile duct as it runs through that viscus, (2) a gall-stone becomes impacted in the duct, or (3) a stricture develops in the duct, either because of damage by an impacted stone or at previous operation or because of a primary carcinoma of the duct.

Macroscopically, the liver is usually deeply jaundiced and in the later stages the surface may be finely nodular as a result of developing biliary cirrhosis. The cut surface usually shows a very distinct lobular pattern. The bile ducts are markedly dilated above the obstruction.

Microscopically, the liver cells are filled with bile granules, and small globules and cylinders of bile (bile thrombi) appear in canaliculi between adjacent liver cells. In advanced cases large bile-stained foci of necrotic liver cells develop ('bile lakes'). The individual liver cells frequently show degenerative changes. Short stellate fibrous processes usually emanate from the portal tracts which contain an increased number of bile ducts. Inflammatory cells may accumulate in the portal tracts and around necrotic liver cell foci, but they are rarely as numerous as in hepatitis, and, in contrast to the latter, usually include a number of polymorphs. Drugs such as chlorpromazine produce jaundice and give a histological picture very similar to that of early extrahepatic obstruction. This is a hypersensitivity reaction and resolves on withdrawal of the drug. Testosterone produces dose-related obstructive jaundice.

Other liver diseases

Neoplasms

The commonest benign neoplasm (really a congenital malformation) is a cavernous haemangioma which is quite frequently to be observed in a subcapsular position at autopsy. Other hamartomas contain bile ducts. *Metastases* are by far the most frequently observed malignant tumours and these are nearly all carcinomatous. They usually occur as multiple discrete pale-grey nodules and, as the centres are liable to become necrotic, being most distant from the blood supply, those which project on the surface often have depressed centres. Less commonly, the malignant tumours infiltrate diffusely in portal tracts and sinuses so that the neoplastic contour is not so easily seen by the naked eye. The liver may show local chronic venous congestion and cholestasis in the neighbourhood of the nodules. *Primary liver carcinoma* can take two histological forms, one resembling liver cells (hepatoma) and the other bile ducts (cholangiocarcinoma). The nodules are often multiple, and are liable to develop in cirrhotic livers. A rapidly progressive tumour (hepatoblastoma) may arise in infancy and is similar to the commoner primitive tumour of renal origin (nephroblastoma or Wilms' tumour).

The bile

The liver secretes approximately 800 ml of bile per day. It contains bile acids, bile pigments (mainly bilirubin), cholesterol and mucin. The gall bladder concentrates bile four to ten times by absorption of water. Bile salts play an important part in the absorption of fats by emulsifying triglycerides. In this way they also assist in the absorption of calcium and fat-soluble vitamins (A, D and K). They also assist in the activation of proteolytic enzymes. Bile is the main route of excretion of certain metabolites of drugs and hormones, heavy metals, poisons, bile pigment and cholesterol from the body.

Only 80% of the bile pigment is derived from the haemoglobin of broken-down red cells; the remainder comes from an unknown source, probably other haem pigments as in muscle. Haemoglobin breaks down in the reticuloendothelial system to haem and globin; the latter is re-metabolized. The haem forms an iron-containing fraction (haemosiderin) which is conserved by the body, and bilirubin, which is insoluble in water, becoming attached to plasma albumin on its way to the liver. The bilirubin becomes detached from the albumin and conjugated with glucuronic acid in the liver cell, and the resultant water-soluble glucuronide conjugate is passed out into the bile. When the bile reaches the intestine, it is converted by bacteria to stercobilinogen (urobilinogen). Some of this, on oxidation to stercobilin (urobilin), pigments the faeces. The remainder is reabsorbed from the intestine and passes into the liver to be re-excreted. The liver 'threshold' is higher for urobilinogen than for bile, so that when the liver is mildly damaged, or when an excessive load of urobilinogen is presented to it, there is delay in re-excretion of the urobilinogen, and some of the excess passes over into the urine at a time when the liver still excretes bile completely. The renal 'threshold' for albumin-bound bilirubin is much higher than for conjugated glucuronide, with the result that the former never appears in the urine. Most of the conjugated bile acids recirculate via the enterohepatic route, being absorbed in the last 100 cm of ileum.

Jaundice

This is the yellow coloration which results from increased amounts of bile pigments in the body (Fig. 2). Jaundice can result from (1) increased production of bilirubin, as in haemolytic anaemias, (2) impaired uptake of bilirubin into the hepatic parenchymal cells, as is seen in some forms of Gilbert's syndrome (benign familial unconjugated hyperbilirubinaemia), (3) failure of conjugation of bilirubin within the parenchymal cells (e.g. other forms of Gilbert's syndrome, the Crigler–Najjar syndromes and the 'physiological jaundice' of premature infants), (4) failure of excretion of bilirubin into the canaliculi, as is seen in the Dubin–Johnson syndrome, (5) intrahepatic obstruction at the canalicular level (e.g. with anabolic steroid therapy), or at bile duct level (e.g. in primary biliary cirrhosis), (6) extrahepatic obstruction due to gall-stones or tumours of the pancreas.

In the commonest clinical forms of jaundice (hepatocellular disease or obstruction), the defects may be multiple. For example, in hepatocellular disease due to viral hepatitis, decreased uptake, conjugation and excretion occur, sometimes with an element of intrahepatic cholestasis. In an obstructive jaundice due to carcinoma of the pancreas, obstruction will predominate but hepatocellular defects may occur as the liver becomes damaged by the obstruction.

The gall bladder

Gall-stones

Gall-stones are extremely common, being found in about a quarter of all routine post-mortems in Britain, and are much commoner in women than in men. The precise mechanisms leading to their development are still largely obscure; the old-established concept that most stones develop through infection is not proven. They arise through the precipitation of some of the main ingredients of bile—bile pigment, cholesterol, and calcium salts—either because one or more of these components is in excess, or because there is altered absorption by the gall bladder of water and some of the other constituents of the bile. There are three well-recognized types.

1. *Mixed stones*. These are much the commonest and most important clinically. They are faceted, always multiple, and are composed of a mixture of bile pigment, cholesterol, calcium salts, and a protein matrix derived from the lining epithelium. They are shiny and deep greenish-brown, the surface frequently being harder than the core which is laminated and shows varying pigmentation. The gall bladders containing them are usually the seat of chronic inflammation.

2. *Pigment stones*. These stones are multiple, small, hard, rounded or

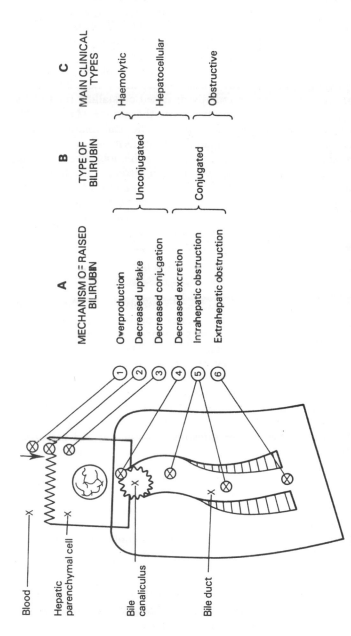

Fig. 2. Different types of jaundice. The diagram shows a parenchymal cell with a bile canaliculus, leading into a bile duct. *Column A* indicates sites where a defect can lead to a build-up in bilirubin. *Column B* indicates whether conjugated or unconjugated bilirubin rises in the plasma as a result of a defect at that site. *Column C* indicates where the lesions are in the clinical types of jaundice. It must be remembered, however, that an obstructive element may develop in hepatocellular disease and also that hepatocellular damage occurs as a result of obstruction.

nodular, and sometimes exist in the form of sand. They are black or dark green in colour, being composed chiefly of bile pigments, with a matrix of organic material and a variable amount of calcium. They occur when the amount of bile pigment is relatively high and therefore develop mainly in cases of long-standing haemolytic anaemia.

3. *Cholesterol stones.* These stones are usually single, averaging 1–2 cm in diameter, are pale brown in colour, finely nodular on the surface, and on section show a radially disposed crystalline texture. A shell of calcium pigment may be deposited on the surface when the gall bladders are inflamed (*combination stone*). The gall bladders may frequently, however, be thin walled, and the mucous membrane studded with fine creamy flecks, due to the presence of histiocytes containing fatty material (cholesterosis or 'strawberry' gall bladder). Cholesterol is held in solution in the bile by the bile acids, and any factor which tends to increase the concentration of cholesterol or decrease that of the bile acids will favour the formation of these stones. Examples are, for the former, obesity, high-fat diet, diabetes and pregnancy, for the latter, inflammation of the gall bladder wall, bile stasis and liver disease.

Natural history

The clinical manifestations of gall bladder disease are mainly the result of the development of gall-stones. Gall-stones tend to be silent clinically unless they migrate into the neck of the gall bladder or into the common bile duct. In the former case, the retained bile may lead to irritation of the gall bladder wall and secondary infection giving *acute or chronic cholecystitis*. If the infection is more severe, the gall bladder may become gangrenous and perforate or result in an empyema of the gall bladder. Inflammation may lead to the formation of fistulae into surrounding structures, notably the small intestine. Large stones passing through these fistulae may, rarely, cause intestinal obstruction and gall-stone ileus. Obstruction to the neck of the gall bladder results in absorption of pigment from the retained bile and accumulation of mucus—a mucocele of the gall bladder. Most examples of carcinoma of the gall bladder develop in those containing stones and showing changes of chronic cholecystitis. The passage of gall-stones down the common bile duct may be silent or may produce symptoms of pain with intermittent obstructive jaundice. If unrelieved, this may give ascending cholangitis and biliary cirrhosis.

Acute cholecystitis

This, in isolation, is relatively uncommon. It is more frequently seen as a result of obstruction of the cystic duct. There is evidence that the inflammation is initially not bacterial, for in the early period the bile is sterile. However, after 24 hours, infection is superimposed on the chemical inflammation. Macroscopically the gall bladder shows all the features of acute inflammation with ulceration of the mucous membrane and the development of pus in the bile. Necrosis and perforation may result in peritonitis.

Chronic cholecystitis

This is much more commonly observed. The gall bladder is shrunken and pale grey, with fibrous adhesions on the surface. On section, the wall is greatly thickened, and the mucous membrane pale olive-green, pitted and somewhat velvety. Microscopically, the normal papillary mucous membrane is considerably flattened and may be absent in places. There is a great increase of fibrous tissue in the wall, chiefly located outside the muscle coat. A variable amount of chronic inflammatory cell infiltration is present. The mucous membrane is liable to herniate through the loose muscularis to form the so-called Rokitansky–Aschoff sinuses. These may ulcerate, and the bile in the lumen may thus add to the chronic inflammatory reaction in the wall. The arteries in the wall show evidence of endarteritis obliterans.

Gall-stone impaction in the common duct

This is the commonest cause of extrahepatic biliary obstruction, and the jaundice is classically associated with pain, with or without intermittent fever. In a proportion of cases, however, the jaundice is symptomless. The bile duct is dilated above the obstruction. In a minority of cases, acute purulent inflammation of the proximal branches may develop (acute cholangitis). Stones impacted in the ampulla of Vater may be associated with acute pancreatitis.

Tumours of the gall bladder and bile ducts

Papillary adenomas may occasionally develop in the gall bladder. Carcinomas form about 1% of all malignant tumours. They occur mostly either at the fundus or the neck and tend to infiltrate locally into the adjacent liver. Metastases to the regional lymph nodes are common. Most are adenocarcinomas of varying differentiation but sometimes metaplastic squamous carcinomas develop. Carcinomas of the bile duct are of the same order of frequency; they are also adenocarcinomas and either cause stricture of a main duct or present as an intrahepatic tumour.

The pancreas

Diabetes mellitus

Diabetes mellitus is the name given to a group of conditions in which metabolic abnormalities such as hyperglycaemia are associated with a relative lack of insulin, and in which chronic complications develop, usually associated with microvascular lesions. The two major forms are juvenile and maturity-onset diabetes. In the former, control of the blood glucose is usually insulin dependent, but in the latter, oral antidiabetic agents and diet are usually effective. The major life-threatening acute complication is hyperglycaemic coma. This is usually associated with ketoacidosis in the juvenile group and with hyperosmolar coma in the maturity-onset cases. Hypoglycaemic coma is a complication of treatment, i.e. too much insulin. The chronic complications are many and various. Capillary basement membrane thickening occurs in many organs and atheroma is more marked in diabetes; ischaemic lesions such as infarcts are therefore more common. Retinopathy, based on a vascular abnormality, occurs and may lead to blindness. Renal complications include nodular glomerulosclerosis (Kimmelstiel–Wilson lesion), and glomerular basement membrane thickening may be associated with a nephrotic syndrome. Papillary necrosis, pyelonephritis and ischaemic damage can all contribute to the renal failure which commonly occurs. Whether close control of the blood glucose prevents all these complications is an issue which is still debated.

The pancreas is usually normal macroscopically and in over half the cases the islets appear normal microscopically. In the rest there are varying degrees of hyalinization of the islets, hydropic degeneration of the cells and in some cases there is lymphocytic infiltration of the islets. A direct cause of diabetes is known in only a few cases, such as when the islets are destroyed in haemochromatosis or by extensive tumour. In the juvenile-onset type there is good evidence (family studies, HLA groups) that hereditary factors are important and that viral infection can lead to immune destruction of the islets in some cases. Maturity onset diabetes also shows hereditary factors.

Tumours of the pancreas

Carcinoma of the exocrine portion of the pancreas is common, being responsible for about 5% of all tumour deaths in Britain. Such carcinomas occur more frequently in males and are seen in middle-aged and elderly people. Three-quarters of them occur in the head of the pancreas so that obstruction to the pancreatic and common bile ducts easily occurs, often producing jaundice, pain, pancreatitis and anaemia due to bleeding. The tumour spreads directly into other organs but also via lymphatics, the bloodstream and the peritoneal cavity, and may present with the effects of a metastasis. Tumours in the tail are particularly likely to present with a non-metastatic syndrome, such as fleeting thrombophlebitis or a pyrexia of unknown origin. Macroscopically, the carcinoma usually forms a hard pale-grey nodule with ill-defined borders. Microscopically, the nodules are adenocarcinomas of varying degrees of differentiation.

Tumours of the endocrine portion of the pancreas are much less common. They produce their effects mainly by hormone production. An insulinoma (β-cell tumour) produces hypoglycaemic attacks. A gastrinoma results in the Zollinger–Ellison syndrome with high gastric acid secretion and severe peptic ulceration. Glucagon, somatostatin and vasoactive intestinal polypeptide (VIP) production by islet cell tumours have all been reported but are rare. Histologically, all these tumours look like carcinoid tumours and a true carcinoid, producing serotonin, may occur. Many islet cell tumours are benign, some are multiple, some invade and metastasize.

Pancreatitis

This may occur in acute and chronic forms. *Acute interstitial pancreatitis* develops as a complication of mumps, but little is known of the microscopical lesion in this instance, as nearly all cases recover spontaneously. *Acute haemorrhagic pancreatitis* is a well-recognized cause of an acute abdominal emergency, which is much more frequently diagnosed than substantiated. It is brought about by digestion of the organ and surrounding peritoneal fatty tissue by its own powerful enzymes. The mechanism of the release of the enzymes is obscure, but appears to be associated with a rise in intraductular pressure. There may be a gall-stone impacted in the ampulla of Vater or there may be a stricture of the pancreatic duct. Attacks frequently follow large meals and are more common in alcoholics. Less commonly, the initiating factor may be vascular, either atheroma or polyarteritis nodosa, causing ischaemic necrosis of the gland and release of digestive enzymes. The pancreas is swollen and haemorrhagic. Creamy yellow flecks of fat necrosis may be seen in the surrounding fat. Microscopically, the pancreas is largely autolysed and areas of haemorrhage are present with some exudation of polymorph leucocytes. The latter are usually few in number as most of the inflammation and necrosis is chemical. High levels of serum amylase confirm the diagnosis. Acute pancreatitis is a serious disease with a high mortality. A few cases recover but they may be left with a pseudocyst of the pancreas consisting of incompletely organized blood clot and fat necrosis. *Chronic pancreatitis* is another disease of obscure aetiology. It appears to follow repeated minor attacks of acute pancreatitis and is particularly associated with alcoholism. Some cases may also follow obstruction of the pancreatic duct or ampulla of Vater by carcinoma or calculus. The pancreas feels diffusely firm or hard and may suggest carcinoma. The histological picture is one of glandular atrophy, initially with surviving islets of Langerhans, but later these also atrophy, to be replaced by fibrous tissue. There may be infiltration of the gland by chronic inflammatory cells. Haemochromatosis (see p. 164) may also give diffuse fibrosis of the pancreas, but this is associated with heavy deposition of iron.

Cystic fibrosis

Cystic fibrosis produces a pathological picture in the pancreas similar to that of chronic pancreatitis except that the surviving ducts are usually cystic and contain inspissated mucin. This forms part of a systemic disease involving mucus secretion in ducts in the pancreas, lungs and liver; it also involves sweat glands and salivary glands. The disease is more appropriately referred to as *mucoviscidosis*. It is an autosomal recessive and occurs in about 1/1600 of Caucasian births. In neonatal life it may present as intestinal obstruction due to inspissated meconium in the gut—meconium ileus. Later, it becomes manifest as malabsorption due to pancreatic failure. These children also develop bronchiectasis with recurrent respiratory infections, and chronic biliary obstruction leading to cirrhosis. There is excessive secretion of sodium and chloride by sweat glands and salivary glands. The disease is considered by some to be due to an abnormality of mucolytic enzymes, but others regard it as due to an abnormal mucin.

Pancreatic cysts

Retention cysts in the pancreas may be associated with duct obstruction as found in mucoviscidosis. *Congenital cysts* are usually larger, and lined by duct epithelium; there may also be cysts in the kidney and liver. *Pseudocysts* do not have an epithelial lining; they consist of old blood and cellular debris surrounded by fibrous tissue, the result of previous acute haemorrhagic pancreatitis or trauma. *Neoplastic cysts* may be benign or malignant. These cystadenomas and cystadenocarcinomas are mucus secreting and are similar to the corresponding mucinous cysts in the ovary.

18

The Urinary Tract

The kidneys

Renal disease produces clinical effects mainly as a result of (a) functional failure, (b) hypertension, (c) infection, and (d) malignant disease.

Common manifestations of impaired renal function include the following.

1. *Asymptomatic proteinuria*, detected on routine examination of urine, results from increased permeability of the glomerular basement membrane.

2. *Nephrotic syndrome*: when urinary protein loss is severe, i.e. in excess of 5 g/24 h in an adult, this syndrome of proteinuria, hypoalbuminaemia and oedema occurs. Hypercholesterolaemia is often present.

3. *Recurrent haematuria* may exist without other functional effects.

4. *Acute nephritic syndrome*—haematuria, oliguria, oedema, hypertension and retention of nitrogenous products.

5. *Renal failure* is a reduction in glomerular filtration rate sufficient to cause substantial alteration in plasma biochemistry. Acute renal failure develops in days (or weeks) but chronic renal failure develops in months (or years). 'Uraemia' covers all features associated with renal failure. Diseases causing renal failure may remain symptomless until a very advanced stage, but then the manifestations include anorexia, nausea, vomiting, thirst, hiccoughs, itching, anaemia, hypertension, pericarditis, pericardial effusion, pulmonary oedema, renal osteodystrophy and disturbances of cerebral and peripheral nerve function. The cause of renal failure may be intrinsic renal disease but also may be pre-renal (e.g. vascular insufficiency) or post-renal (e.g. urinary tract obstruction).

6. *Hypertension* and its effects.

Glomerulonephritis

This term covers a group of disorders in which the primary lesion in the kidney is in the glomeruli. The glomerulonephritis may be 'isolated' ('primary') or may be part of a systemic disease (e.g. bacterial endocarditis). Because the different forms of glomerulonephritis vary in aetiology, pathogenesis, treatment and prognosis, it is necessary to classify them into subgroups. The most useful classification to date is that based on morphology of glomeruli by light microscopy.

Classification

1. Minimal change.
2. Membranous.
3. Proliferative
   a. Diffuse: acute exudative, crescentic, mesangial, membrano-proliferative
   b. Focal.
4. Sclerotic: focal and segmental sclerosis.
5. End-stage and unclassifiable.

Minimal change glomerulonephritis tends to occur in childhood producing proteinuria and the nephrotic syndrome. It is usually associated with a highly selective proteinuria (i.e. small molecules of albumin escape through the glomerular capillary walls but the larger globulin molecules are retained in the circulation) and responds to steroids, though it may relapse. The glomeruli look normal on light microscopy but fusion of the foot processes of the podocytes is seen with electron microscopy. No immunoglobulins are fixed in the glomeruli.

Membranous glomerulonephritis produces proteinuria, the nephrotic syndrome and ultimately impairment of renal function. The proteinuria is not selective and does not usually respond to steroids. Patients tend to remit and relapse over many years, eventually developing chronic renal failure. The glomeruli have normal cellularity and thickened but abnormally leaky basement membranes. Electron microscopy shows subepithelial deposits with 'spikes' of basement membrane between them. Immunofluorescence shows that these deposits contain IgG and complement.

Proliferative glomerulonephritis is the group which gives the most difficulty in understanding but, as some patterns are associated with complete recovery while others lead inexorably and rapidly to renal failure, it is important to try to distinguish them. The diffuse forms involve all glomeruli. In *acute exudative glomerulonephritis*, endothelial and mesangial cell proliferation is associated with a polymorph infiltrate; subepithelial humps are seen on electron microscopy, and granular immunoglobulin and complement deposits are usually present in glomeruli. The proliferation leads to obliteration of the glomerular capillaries, reduced glomerular filtration, and impairment of tubular function. This process underlies many of the cases of acute nephritic syndrome of childhood and adult life, though other clinical presentations are possible. Provided death does not occur in the acute phase, there is complete recovery in most cases.

Crescentic glomerulonephritis may have similar clinical features but microscopy shows epithelial proliferation within Bowman's capsule, giving the appearance of 'crescents' in more than 70% of glomeruli. Rapidly advancing renal failure is the rule, so that the prognosis of this form is very bad, with few cases retaining enough renal function to sustain life two years after diagnosis.

The two other forms of diffuse proliferative glomerulonephritis may present in various ways and tend to be associated with gradual impairment of function, which is usually much slower in pure *mesangial proliferation* than with the *membranoproliferative* form, where basement membrane abnormalities are also apparent. Pure mesangial cell proliferation may be associated with IgA deposition and recurrent haematuria (Berger's nephropathy).

In focal proliferative glomerulonephritis, where only some glomeruli show proliferation (and this is often segmental, i.e. involving only parts of the glomerulus), a systemic disorder such as bacterial endocarditis or systemic lupus erythematosus is often involved and should always be sought. The prognosis is that of the underlying disorder.

The forms which progress give rise to sclerotic hyalinized glomeruli and in this *end-stage* it is virtually impossible to diagnose the original pattern. One form, focal sclerosing glomerulonephritis with hyalinosis, appears to be sclerotic *ab initio*, with virtually no proliferation. It tends to present with proteinuria or nephrotic syndrome, giving a non-selective proteinuria resistant to steroids and progressing to renal failure.

In end-stage renal failure, the kidneys are small and finely scarred with a thin cortex and blurring of the corticomedullary junctions. The glomeruli are sclerotic, the tubules mainly atrophic, and interstitial tissue increased in amount. The arteries and arterioles often show hypertensive changes.

Aetiology and pathogenesis

Most cases are believed to have an immunological basis. Experiments have shown two models that have human equivalents. Circulating antibody to glomerular basement membrane results in a proliferative glomerulonephritis with linear deposition of immunoglobulin along the membrane: this is a rare form of human disease but is found in Goodpasture's syndrome (Type II hypersensitivity) where pulmonary haemorrhage is associated with proliferative glomerulonephritis. In immune complex disease (Type III hypersensitivity), circulating antigen–antibody complexes become fixed in the glomerular capillary wall or may unite at this site to produce granular immunoglobulin deposits which activate complement and, in some cases, results in inflammation; this pattern of immunoglobulin deposition is often seen in human disease, in membranous and usually in proliferative glomerulonephritis. Antigens which have been incriminated in the aetiology of glomerulonephritis include some associated with infectious organisms (e.g. haemolytic streptococci with acute exudative glomerulonephritis, *Plasmodium malariae* with nephrotic syndrome) and others such as DNA and tumour antigens. The nature of the host response is probably more important than the presence of a particular antigen in determining the outcome. Other mechanisms (known and unknown) are also involved.

Glomerulonephritis is seen in many *systemic diseases*, especially those involving immune reactions (e.g. systemic lupus erythematosus and polyarteritis nodosa). It may not be possible to see specific changes in the kidney, only an appearance which suggests the diagnosis. An exception is in SLE, where haematoxyphil bodies (corresponding to the inclusions of LE cells) are diagnostic. Some systemic diseases produce glomerular changes which are not usually regarded as glomerulonephritis. Amyloid, for example, when deposited in the glomeruli, results in proteinuria and the nephrotic syndrome. Diabetes mellitus may be associated with a nodular glomerulosclerosis (Kimmelstiel–Wilson lesion) or with a diffuse thickening of the basement membranes—both lesions producing proteinuria.

Renal biopsy is often performed in adults in order to discover the type of glomerular lesion causing clinical disease. In children the lesions are more predictable, for the nephrotic syndrome is almost always due to minimal change disease and the acute nephritic syndrome usually to an acute exudative glomerulonephritis. Treatment of these children is therefore started without doing a biopsy. It is only when they fail to follow the predicted course that a biopsy is performed.

Pyelonephritis

This has been an overdiagnosed condition. It originally implied an infection of the pelvis and renal parenchyma which passed through an acute phase to become chronic, leading to a coarsely scarred kidney with hypertension and renal failure. Overdiagnosis occurred because of the assumption that all coarsely scarred kidneys were infective in origin, but such an interstitial nephritis may result from analgesic abuse, vascular changes, or irradiation. Chronic pyelonephritis does occur on an infective basis, but is almost always associated with an urinary tract abnormality; *Escherichia coli* is the commonest organism involved. In acute pyelonephritis the pelvis of the kidney is congested and, later, purulent streaks can be seen to radiate from it into the medulla and cortex. Abscesses may develop. In chronic pyelonephritis changes are similar to those of ischaemia. The kidneys are reduced in size, showing coarse scarring, loss of cortical tissue and blurring of corticomedullary demarcation. The pelvicalyceal architecture is also distorted. Histology shows glomerulosclerosis, periglomerular fibrosis, tubular atrophy, interstitial inflammation and arterial changes of hypertension. The dilated tubules contain protein casts. The renal pelvis also shows chronic inflammation. If the infection is active, polymorph leucocyte infiltration of tubules and interstitium can be seen.

Papillary necrosis

This is an important complication of analgesic abuse over many years. There is avascular necrosis of the renal papillae which are shed in the urine, giving rise to impaired renal function. Papillary necrosis may also be a complication of acute pyelonephritis, especially when this complicates diabetes mellitus or urinary obstruction.

Renal tuberculosis

The organ becomes infected by way of the bloodstream and progressive disease more frequently involves one kidney than both. It may be a complication of miliary tuberculosis, in which case the small grey nodules can be seen throughout the renal parenchyma or a focal caseating lesion may be found. Focal lesions usually arise near the corticomedullary junction but spread to involve the renal pelvis giving tuberculous pyelonephritis. Obstruction to the ureter by granulomatous inflammation leads to tuberculous pyonephrosis. The histological features are typical of tuberculous granulomas. The lesions may heal, leaving fibrous or calcified scars. Tuberculous pyonephrosis may destroy the whole renal parenchyma leaving a fibrous renal capsule surrounding caseous material—autonephrectomy. Infection commonly spreads to involve the ureter, bladder, prostate and epididymis.

Hydronephrosis

Hydronephrosis is dilatation of the renal pelvis with some atrophy of renal parenchyma. It is caused by chronic partial obstruction to urinary flow and may be unilateral or bilateral. Unilateral hydronephrosis is usually associated with ureteric obstruction which may be due to malformation of the pelvi-ureteric junction, or it may follow scarring of the surrounding tissues, tumour in the wall, or calculus in the lumen. Bilateral hydronephrosis may be due to external pressure on the ureters associated with tumour or retroperitoneal fibrosis; it may be due to tumour of the bladder or to obstruction at the bladder neck (prostatic hypertrophy) or urethra (gonococcal stricture). With increasing degrees of hydronephrosis, the renal parenchyma becomes increasingly stretched and its blood supply increasingly obstructed, so that the nephrons undergo replacement fibrosis. The kidney thus becomes progressively less able to excrete urine and ultimately renal failure follows. This result of urinary obstruction is complicated in many instances by infection (cystitis and pyelonephritis), which is very liable to occur whenever urine becomes stagnant in the urinary tract.

Renal calculi

Common constituents are calcium oxalate, calcium phosphate, magnesium ammonium phosphate and urates, and these salts account for 95% of all stones. Amino-acid stones occur rarely. Calculi develop because of precipation of solutes from the urine. Several factors are known to play a part in stone formation. These include: (1) increase in the amount of solute, e.g. calcium in hyperparathyroidism, uric acid in gout; (2) decrease in the amount of solvent, e.g. dehydration; (3) presence of a nidus acting as a focus for precipitation, e.g. bacteria: (4) urinary obstruction giving stasis and infection; and (5) urea-splitting organisms giving an alkaline urine which is associated with magnesium ammonium phosphate stones. The main effects of stones are obstruction, chronic infection, haematuria and renal colic. They may also be found in the ureter and bladder: bladder stones are much commoner in some underdeveloped countries than in Britain. Calcium oxalate stones are laminated, hard and spiky or nodular. Calcium phosphate stones are larger and chalky, sometimes forming a cast of the renal pelvis (staghorn calculi). Uric-acid stones are usually pale, yellowish and smooth.

Renal cysts

Multiple small cysts are common in any scarred kidney. *Solitary large cysts* are uncommon and seldom cause symptoms. It is when most of the kidney is occupied by cysts that renal impairment occurs. These conditions arise as developmental anomalies. *Congenital polycystic kidney* is the most important group, of which there are two major forms. The most common is the *adult-type* polycystic kidney which is inherited as an autosomal dominant. It does not usually present until adult life, most commonly with haematuria, hypertension, uraemia or an abdominal mass. At this stage the kidneys are massively enlarged and the parenchyma replaced with large, fluid-containing cysts. Cysts may also be present in other organs such as the liver. Another important association is berry aneurysm in the circle of Willis which causes death from subarachnoid haemorrhage in some cases. The *infantile type* is rare and is an autosomal recessive resulting in the kidneys being replaced by countless elongated radially arranged cystic tubules, incompatible with life. Another form of cystic disease is *dysplastic kidney*, which may affect one or both kidneys and may be associated with urinary tract obstruction. This obstruction may itself be a manifestation of dysplasia because similar obstruction may be found simultaneously in the gastrointestinal tract. The pathological characteristics of dysplastic kidney are the presence of malformed tubules, associated with other abnormal tissues such as malformed blood vessels, bone and cartilage.

Cortical necrosis

Bilateral symmetrical cortical necrosis is a rare complication of obstetric shock, endotoxic shock or severe dehydration in infants. The mechanism is not clearly understood but two factors seem to be of importance. There may be shunting of blood through juxtamedullary glomeruli so that the cortex is deprived of blood and there is intravascular thrombosis in small capillaries and arterioles, seen particularly in glomeruli. This thrombosis can be produced experimentally by the repeated intravenous injection of endotoxin (Shwartzman reaction). The cortex is infarcted and there is acute renal failure which does not resolve.

Tubular necrosis

This is more common than cortical necrosis and is seen following renal transplantation, shock, crush injury, poisoning or incompatible blood transfusions. Grossly, the kidneys may be slightly enlarged and pale. Histologically, the lower nephron contains many pigment casts and the lining epithelium is lost. Tubular epithelium may regenerate and if renal biopsies are examined days or weeks after the initial episode, dilated tubules may be found lined by flat, regenerated epithelial cells. At first, patients with tubular necrosis show acute renal failure, but if they can be dialysed in the acute period and the cause removed, then recovery usually follows.

Renal transplantation

This is a successful means of treatment of some cases of chronic renal failure. The ideal donor is a living identical twin, but this is rarely possible. Histocompatibility is therefore a problem and rejection is a common complication, despite immunosuppressive therapy. There are three patterns of rejection, which overlap.

1. *Hyperacute rejection.* In recipients with preformed antibodies to the donor cells, thrombi form in small vessels within a few minutes of transplantation. This leads to rapid infarction of the organ which never functions and has to be removed.
2. *Acute rejection.* Many recipients have an episode of acute rejection in the first few months. Clinically there is fever, oliguria, tender swelling of the graft kidney, increased systemic blood pressure, and proteinuria. Pathologically there are two types:
   a. predominantly cell mediated, where there is oedema and infiltration of the graft with lymphoid cells, and tubular damage;
   b. predominantly humoral, where fibrin, platelets and polymorphs are found in small vessels. When more severe, it resembles hyperacute rejection.

3. *Chronic rejection*. Gradual deterioration of the graft may occur, without a clinical 'rejection episode'. Arterial narrowing by concentric intimal proliferation (probably caused by slow humoral damage) is the most significant lesion. It leads to ischaemia of the graft. Glomerular, tubular and interstitial damage may be seen.

Apart from rejection, many other complications may develop after renal transplantation. Acute tubular necrosis frequently occurs in the immediate postoperative stage but usually resolves. There may be occlusion or rupture of the arterial, venous or ureteric anastamosis. Infection may develop, either in the graft or elsewhere in the immunosuppressed patient. Long term, there is an increased incidence of tumours, particularly lymphomas, in recipients.

Renal tumours

Very small fibromas, leiomyomas and lipomas may be found in the subcapsular cortex but they are not of clinical significance. Tubular adenomas occur most frequently in scarred kidneys. They are usually tiny but if large they may be difficult to distinguish from cortical carcinomas. All tubular tumours over 3 cm diameter should be treated as malignant. A renal hamartoma (angiomyolipoma) may grow to a large size mimicking carcinoma. These are benign tumour-like malformations which may be solitary but can be found in patients with tuberose sclerosis.

Carcinoma of the renal parenchyma (hypernephroma)

This accounts for three-quarters of all malignant tumours of the kidney and about 1% of all malignant diseases. It characteristically consists of a spherical mass at one pole of the kidney and on section presents a mottled red, brown, yellow and grey surface, which is partly cystic. The different colours are due to haemorrhage, necrosis, fibrosis, and accumulation of fat in the tumour. The tumour may extend into the renal vein. Histologically, a tubular pattern is common, and frequently the tumour cells have a characteristic water-clear cytoplasm. An intracystic papillary pattern is another histological variant.

As might be expected from the tendency to extend into the renal vein, bloodstream spread is common, and the lungs, brain, and bones are frequent sites for metastases. Lymph node metastases are found in about one-third of cases.

Tumours of the renal pelvis

These comprise about one-seventh of all renal tumours. Together with those of the ureter, their structure and behaviour are similar to those of the bladder, described below.

Wilms's tumour

Wilms's tumour accounts for the remainder of primary malignant tumours and has been described on p. 76. It rarely occurs outside childhood and is most common in the first five years of life. The tumour is grey or white and infiltrates surrounding structures. Metastases are common both by way of lymphatics and bloodstream.

The urinary bladder

Cystitis

Inflammation of the bladder mucosa giving rise to pain and frequency of micturition is common, especially in women. It is usually bacterial (especially associated with *Escherichia coli*, *Proteus mirabilis* or *Streptococcus faecalis*) but can be associated with other organisms (e.g. *Monilia* or *Schistosoma*) or with other irritants such as heavy metals, drugs or irradiation. Ascending infection is the usual route of entry of bacteria and the shortness of the female urethra is a predisposing factor, as is obstruction to urine outflow; this may give rise to infection anywhere in the urinary tract, for any residual urine after voiding results in infection and the lumen is then never free of bacteria.

In acute cystitis the mucosa is congested, oedematous and has a polymorph infiltrate. If the inflammation becomes chronic, lymphocytes become the predominant inflammatory cell and fibrosis occurs. Sometimes the epithelium dips down, forming small cysts in the wall—*cystitis cystica*. *Interstitial cystitis* (Hunner's ulcer) occurs in middle-aged women and may progress to fibrous contraction of the bladder; it is of unknown aetiology.

Hypertrophy and dilatation

The bladder is capable of considerable hypertophy and dilatation if there is obstruction to urinary outflow in the urethra, as, for example, by prostatic enlargement. It is liable to become dilated if there is loss of nervous control. A hypertrophied but empty bladder has a thickened wall, with well-marked trabeculae on its inner surface. Sometimes obstruction to urinary outflow may lead to the formation of a diverticulum in the bladder wall which is liable to ulcerate and may perforate.

Tumours

The vast majority of bladder tumours are carcinomas or papillomas. They account for about 3% of deaths from all forms of malignant disease. The incidence of bladder carcinoma is greater in men than in women and it appears to be increasing. There is a recognized association with exposure to certain chemicals in industry. These include aniline dyes, benzidene, β-naphthylamine and 4-amino-diphenyl, formerly used as an antioxidant in the rubber and plastics industry. Metabolites of tryptophan are related to naphthylamine and may account for some non-industrial carcinomas. There is a higher incidence in patients with schistosomiasis, but this may be the result of chronic inflammation of the bladder rather than a direct carcinogenic effect of the parasite. Squamous carcinoma is found in diverticula of the bladder. Congenital defect of the bladder and abdominal wall leaves the posterior surface of the bladder exposed (exstrophy) and this gives rise to chronic inflammation in which adenocarcinomas may develop.

Most tumours of the bladder recur and eventually infiltrate the underlying wall. Few are therefore 'benign' and the term *papilloma* is confined to less than 5% of papillary tumours in which the mucosa of the papillary folds is not heaped up or irregular and there is no invasion. *Carcinomas* are either papillary or solid in shape, the latter having a worse prognosis. Most are differentiated *transitional cell carcinomas*, but metaplasia is common and squamous carcinoma or adenocarcinoma is also found. Anaplastic carcinoma and adenocarcinoma may be difficult to distinguish from secondary carcinoma infiltrating the bladder. Primary carcinomas remain confined to the mucosa for some time, but eventually infiltrate the muscle coat and perivesical tissues. Metastases to pelvic and para-aortic lymph nodes and by bloodstream to liver and lungs occur late.

In children, *embryonal rhabdomyosarcoma* may occur in the bladder. This is a rare tumour which is highly malignant and grows in a grape-like fashion in the lumen (botryoid sarcoma). The same type of tumour is found in the cervix and vagina of girls.

19

The Male Genital Tract

The prostate

Benign enlargement or hyperplasia

Benign prostatic hyperplasia is a very common change in the prostate of elderly men. It is sometimes called myoadenoma, but this is not an acceptable term as the abnormality does not consist of a single nodule, but of an irregularly distributed overgrowth in the gland. It is considered to result from the endocrine imbalance which occurs at that period of life.

When examined with the naked eye, the prostate may show considerable enlargement of much of the gland or the overgrowth may be limited to one part. The change does not affect the posterior portion of the gland. The lateral lobes of the anterior portion may be mainly involved, but frequently a striking feature is a polypoid swelling of the median lobe which projects into the bladder cavity, exerting a flap-valve effect on the flow of urine through the prostatic urethra. The swelling of the lateral lobes also stretches and kinks the urethra, so it is not surprising that the major complication of this disease is retention of urine. On section, ill-defined vesicular or solid nodules are present in the fibrous stroma. Milky fluid exudes from the vesicles.

On histological examination, the nodules can be seen to consist mainly of a great overgrowth of the prostatic glandular epithelium, the supporting fibromuscular tissue growing pari passu. The epithelial cells in some glands become atrophic. Occasional nodules consist of smooth muscle and fibrous tissue only. Small infarcts sometimes develop, and there is variable chronic inflammation.

The main complications of prostatic enlargement are acute or chronic retention of urine with or without superadded infection.

Carcinoma

Prostatic adenocarcinoma accounts for 7% of all tumour deaths in males. It mainly starts in the posterior lobes so it is often felt on rectal examination. Diagnosis is made by biopsy.

Prostatic carcinoma presents clinically because of urinary obstruction, or because of local infiltration outside the gland, or because of metastasis. It spreads via the lymphatics and bloodstream and is particularly likely to give metastases in bones, which are usually osteosclerotic. A raised serum acid phosphatase is often present. Microscopic foci of carcinoma are found in prostates at post-mortem much more commonly than clinically active carcinomas are seen. It is customary, therefore, to classify prostatic carcinomas according to their biological behaviour; most are adenocarcinomas. *Clinical carcinomas* are those which are producing symptoms (either from obstruction or from metastases) and are readily detected in the gland. *Occult carcinomas* are those which present as metastases but where the primary lesion is elusive. *Latent carcinomas* are those microscopic foci which have all the histological features of carcinoma within the gland but which have not produced symptoms and have not metastasized. Pathological methods are not, as yet, good enough to predict which latent tumours will become biologically active, but lack of differentiation is associated with an aggressive behaviour. Oestrogens may cause involution of the carcinoma but the tumour is not eradicated by this treatment.

Inflammation

Acute prostatitis is rare. It usually develops as a result of infection in the bladder or posterior urethra or it may follow surgery and instrumentation. Chronic prostatitis leading to the formation of a hard, shrunken prostate, often containing a number of small calculi, may be the result of gonococcal infection or it may be due to coliform organisms. Granulomatous prostatitis is seen in tuberculous infections. The prostate is affected in about three-quarters of the cases of genitourinary tuberculosis. Cavitating caseating granulomas may eventually destroy much of the gland. Non-specific granulomatous prostatitis produces a histological picture very similar to that of tuberculosis but acid-fast bacilli are not found. This reaction is caused by rupture of prostatic ducts, often as a result of inflammation or obstruction due to benign hyperplasia. The released secretion initiates the tuberculoid granulomas. The gland becomes fibrotic and hard, and is frequently mistaken clinically for carcinoma.

Urethra and penis

Acute urethritis is usually venereal and may be gonococcal or non-gonococcal in origin. In the male, *Neisseria gonorrhoeae* gives rise to a suppurative inflammation in the mucosa of the urethra. Sometimes epididymitis occurs and the infection may become disseminated but usually responds quickly to antibiotics. Neglected cases may result in urethral stricture.

Many cases of non-gonococcal urethritis are due to *Chlamydia trachomatis* and may show a range of clinical manifestations similar to those of gonococcal infections. *Reiter's syndrome* consists of arthritis, urethritis, conjunctivitis and mucocutaneous lesions; the HLA-B27 antigen is common in these patients; there may also be urethritis associated with chlamydia.

Primary syphilis develops as a chancre, usually on the glans penis or prepuce, two to six weeks after infection. At first it is an indurated papule which breaks down to form a punched-out ulcer. The chronic inflammatory infiltrate contains many plasma cells and there is endarteritis of the small vessels around the ulcer. It heals to leave a fibrous scar. *Secondary syphilis* may involve the penis, scrotum and perianal skin, causing warty growths (condylomata lata) in which spirochaetes are numerous.

Lymphogranuloma venereum is an infection with certain invasive strains of *Chlamydia trachomatis* which give rise to a granulomatous inflammation in pelvic and inguinal lymph nodes, leading to lymphatic obstruction. It is usually acquired venereally (and is commoner in the Tropics) but the primary lesion on the penis often escapes detection.

Granuloma inguinale is rare in Britain, though endemic in the Tropics. The primary lesion on the penis is a spreading ulcer with surrounding chronic inflammation in which histiocytes, containing Donovan bodies, can be seen. These are bacteria, similar to *Klebsiella* but identified as *Calymmatobacterium granulomatis*, which cause the disease. Involvement of inguinal lymph nodes causes sinuses and scarring.

Tumours

Urethral tumours are rare. Transitional cell carcinomas may develop in the posterior urethra but in the penile urethra they are more commonly squamous carcinomas and occur near the meatus. Carcinoma of the penis is rare in Britain but in parts of Africa and Asia it is one of the commonest forms of malignant disease. It presents on the glans or inner aspect of the prepuce as a fungating mass of squamous carcinoma. It metastasizes to inguinal lymph nodes. Premalignant dysplasia, similar to that in the cervix, may be seen in the penile skin before invasive carcinoma develops. Squamous carcinoma of the scrotum was known as 'chimney-sweeps' cancer' due to the carcinogenic effect of soot in this industry. It is still more common in town dwellers and in those working with tar.

The testis

Miscellaneous disorders

Cystic swellings are common in association with the testis. A hydrocele is due to the accumulation of fluid within the tunica vaginalis, the wall of which is usually thickened by fibrous tissue and may contain a few inflammatory cells. While some hydroceles may be a consequence of inflammation, the aetiology of most remains obscure. Cysts may also develop in association with the epididymis. These are lined by flattened epithelium and contain clear fluid in which spermatozoa may be identified, for which reason they are often called *spermatoceles*. The testis may become infected (*orchitis*). Mumps orchitis is a painful affliction complicating the parotitis in the adolescent or adult, and may cause infertility when there is bilateral testicular involvement. Acute bacterial orchitis is relatively rare but may follow prostatectomy. Tuberculosis may involve the testis by way of the bloodstream or from the urinary tract. The infection usually starts in the epididymis and spreads from there into the body of the testis. In advanced cases the vas deferens and seminal vesicles may become infected. Gumma of the testis was an important differential diagnosis from malignant tumour in the days when tertiary syphilis was common. Syphilis can also cause a diffuse interstitial orchitis.

The spermatic cord may undergo spontaneous *torsion*, resulting in venous infarction of the testis. Atrophy of the testes, whether due to primary testicular failure or as a result of pituitary failure, commonly results in sterility. Varying degrees of testicular atrophy are also associated with undescended testes in the adult and with the chromosomal abnormality of *Klinefelter's syndrome* (see p. 61). In undescended testes there is atrophy of the germinal epithelium of the seminiferous tubules, thickening of the tubular basement membrane and often an apparent increase in number of the interstitial cells.

Tumours

Primary tumours of the testis are uncommon and may arise from testicular parenchymal cells or supporting elements. Primary malignant tumours (mainly germ cell tumours—seminomas and teratomas) account for about 0.3% of all malignant tumour deaths in the male. Their peak incidence is in young and middle-aged men, an age distribution different from that of most malignant tumours.

Seminoma arises from the germ cells of the tubules. Undescended testes have ten times the expected incidence. It usually presents as a testicular mass with a peak incidence in the fifth decade. The cut surface usually shows a smooth, homogeneous, greyish mass. Histologically, there are sheets of spheroidal cells, often with interspersed lymphocytes. If left, it metastasizes to the para-aortic lymph nodes. Modern treatment has radically improved prognosis and the five-year survival of a treated tumour apparently confined to the testis is now better than 90%.

Teratomas are a little less common than seminoma and have a peak incidence in the fourth decade. They are also germ cell tumours but are much more variable in their behaviour than seminoma. They consist of embryonic tissues such as bone, cartilage, squamous and glandular epithelia with or without extraembryonic tissues such as trophoblast and yolk sac elements. Prognosis may be indicated by histological appearances which range from differentiated, through intermediate, to undifferentiated. The last-mentioned behave very badly, but even the best-differentiated versions may metastasize, so that a guarded prognosis is always given. If extraembryonic elements (trophoblastic or yolk sac) are present, aggressive behaviour is anticipated. The trophoblastic cells (choriocarcinoma) may secrete human chorionic gonadotrophin and yolk sac tumours produce α-fetoprotein. These tumour markers may be detected in blood and urine and can be used in diagnosis and monitoring. Teratomas metastasize particularly by the bloodstream, but also by lymphatics.

Seminomas and teratomas may occur together as a *combined tumour*.

Interstitial cell (Leydig cell) tumours and *Sertoli cell* tumours occur very rarely and are not usually malignant. *Malignant lymphoma* may occur in the testis as part of a generalized disease but occasionally as a primary lymphoma involving this organ.

Tumours of the cord may cause scrotal swellings. These paratesticular tumours are mainly of connective tissue origin and include lipomas, fibromas, myomas and their malignant counterparts.

20

The Female Genital Tract

Vulva, vagina and cervix

Sexually transmitted diseases cause many lesions in this area. *Herpes virus* (usually type II) causes an ulcerative vulvitis and may also involve the vagina and cervix. The primary lesions are seen most often in young adults and the initial lesion is an intraepithelial bulla; ulceration with secondary inflammation often precedes healing. However, the virus also travels in the sensory nerves to the posterior root ganglia, where it may remain inert until reactivation leads to another crop of lesions on the vulva.

The small primary lesion of *lymphogranuloma venereum* (see p. 187) develops on the vulva up to a month after infection. This usually heals but is followed by a suppurative inguinal lymphadenitis. Extensive pelvic lesions develop in some patients, with sinuses, fistulae, granulation tissue and fibrosis.

Gonorrhoea (*Neisseria gonorrhoeae*) is frequently asymptomatic in the female, though cervicitis, salpingitis, urethritis and Bartholin's gland abscess can all occur.

Granuloma inguinale (see p. 187) causes vulval nodules which ulcerate, the infection spreading to involve other parts of the genital tract and the inguinal lymph nodes. The inflammation shows abundant granulation tissue, with histiocytes containing rod-shaped organisms ('Donovan bodies').

The chancre (the primary lesion of *syphilis*) is commoner on the vulva and cervix, the vagina being rarely affected. Lesions of the secondary phase also occur, their commonest form in this region being the highly infectious flattish warty lesions called condylomata lata which contain many spirochaetes. Snail-track ulcers also occur. Tertiary manifestations are rare at this site.

Trichomonas vaginalis is a flagellate protozoan causing acute and chronic inflammation in the vagina and cervix. It results in vaginal irritation and discharge. Inflammation is marked in some patients but others become asymptomatic carriers with no signs of inflammation.

Pruritus vulvae is a frequent complaint which in many instances has no organic basis. It may, however, be associated with one of the so-called *vulval dystrophies*. These form a group of conditions characterized by abnormal growth of the stratified squamous epithelium, often accompanied by changes in the underlying connective tissue. Nomenclature has been confused because the same naked-eye appearances may be present with different histological lesions. The confusion is particularly marked with the term 'leucoplakia', which is sometimes used to mean a white plaque of hyperkeratosis but at other times to imply a pre-invasive lesion: the word is therefore best avoided. A current classification of vulval dystrophies is as follows.

1. *Hyperplastic dystrophy*. The lesions appear as white, brown and red plaques. Microscopically, the epidermis shows hyperplasia of the prickle cell layer (acanthosis) and there is often hyperkeratosis.

2. *Lichen sclerosus*. This appears as white plaques, often with parchment-like skin. The malpighian layer is thin, often with some degenerative changes in the basal cells. A characteristic finding is that the upper dermis is hyalinized and lacks elastin fibres. Deep to this layer there is usually a chronic inflammatory cell infiltrate.

3. *Mixed dystrophy*. This occurs when lesions of hyperplastic dystrophy and lichen sclerosus appear together.

Squamous carcinoma of the vulva can arise in any of these forms but seems to be related to the degree of cellular atypia in the epithelium. Carcinoma is likeliest in hyperplastic dystrophies with severe atypia (up to 25% may develop carcinoma) and least likely in lichen sclerosus with no atypia (less than 2% develop carcinoma).

Chronic cervicitis unassociated with specific infections is a common finding and is usually asymptomatic. It is often accompanied by *squamous metaplasia* of the glandular endocervical epithelium. An apparent extension of the columnar epithelium on to the ectocervix may occur at puberty or during pregnancy. This is sometimes called an 'erosion' but is better called 'ectopy' for it is due to a hormonally induced change. The columnar epithelium is damaged in the vaginal environment and may ulcerate; later it undergoes squamous metaplasia. *Cystic dilatation* of endocervical glands is often seen with chronic cervicitis; these mucus-filled cysts are called Nabothian follicles. The usual form of *endocervical polyp* is a benign lesion composed of cystically dilated glands with connective tissue, often covered with metaplastic squamous epithelium.

Carcinoma of the cervix uteri accounts for about 3% of deaths from malignancy in women. Some of these are due to adenocarcinoma of the endocervix, but more than 90% result from squamous carcinoma. Deaths from these tumours are rare before the age of 30, but rise in incidence each decade thereafter. The tumour usually arises near the external os and macroscopically it is nodular, ulcerated and bleeds easily. Local complications dominate the clinical picture for it spreads by direct invasion into the uterus, vagina and parametrium, around the bladder and rectum, reaching the pelvic wall. Lymphatic spread also occurs but blood spread is late. Prognosis depends on the stage of the tumour at diagnosis and the overall five-year survival is 60%.

Early onset of active sexual life and multiplicity of partners are two important factors associated with an increased incidence of cervical carcinoma. The pathogenetic mechanism linking the association has not been elucidated, though there is some evidence implicating chronic virus infection (particularly herpes virus). The invasive tumours arise in the squamous epithelium, near the squamocolumnar junction, and a considerable effort is being made to identify the tumours in a pre-invasive stage so that they can be treated more effectively. This is done by screening asymptomatic women and examining cells exfoliated from the surface of the cervix. These cytological appearances can be used to predict the lesions which may be found in the cervical epithelium. Inflammatory processes can give rise to atypical epithelial changes which do not carry a significant risk of invasive tumour. The changes can be distinguished from the cellular atypia (dysplasia) seen in lesions which carry an increased risk of invasive carcinoma. These have been known as mild, moderate or severe *dysplasia* and *carcinoma-in-situ*, but nowadays, in order to emphasize that they are parts of the same process, they are grouped together under the term *cervical intraepithelial neoplasia* (CIN) and are then graded I, II or III. It is believed that, if CIN grade III is left untreated, up to 70% would develop into invasive carcinomas.

Where a good screening programme is in operation, there is some evidence of a declining death rate from cervical carcinoma. In recent times there has been an increased incidence of pre-invasive lesions, particularly in young women, which makes the screening of asymptomatic women all the more necessary.

The body of the uterus

Uterine curettings

Gynaecological specimens make up about one-third of all those handled by a routine surgical histological laboratory, and a large proportion of them consist of curettings from the endometrium. The main reasons for the submission of curettings are as follows: (1) the diagnosis and treatment of incomplete abortion through the identification of chorionic villi, (2) the diagnosis of carcinoma of the uterine body, (3) the diagnosis of cystic glandular hyperplasia, an index of dysfunctional bleeding, (4) the establishment that ovulation has occurred, as part of the examination for infertility, by the demonstration that the endometrium is in the secretory phase, and (5) the diagnosis of inflammation, particularly genital tuberculosis, by the demonstration of endometrial tubercles in premenstrual curettings.

Curettings reveal the phase of the menstrual cycle with considerable precision. During the first five days of the cycle the endometrium breaks down so that only the basal glands remain. These regenerate surface epithelium and from then until the fourteenth day the glands and stroma proliferate under the influence of oestrogen. Mitoses are numerous, producing elongation of the glands. At ovulation and under the influence of progesterone, subnuclear vacuoles appear in the glandular epithelium; these vacuoles pass to the luminal side of the cell by the nineteenth day. From the twentieth day, secretion appears in the gland lumen. Stromal cells develop more cytoplasm and the stroma becomes compact. From the twenty-fifth day, polymorph leucocytes infiltrate the stroma. In the premenstrual endometrium blood leaks into the stroma and this is followed by constriction of the spiral arteries and breakdown of the endometrium.

Cystic glandular hyperplasia

This hyperplasia of the endometrium occurs with anovulatory menstrual cycles, especially at the menopause. It gives rise to irregular bleeding referred to as metropathia haemorrhagica. Prolonged oestrogen stimulation causes excessive endometrial proliferation resulting in a thickened spongy endometrium. Histologically, the glands are cystic and lined by stratified epithelium. With fluctuation in the oestrogen level, pseudomenstrual breakdown occurs, often accompanied by heavy bleeding resulting in iron deficiency anaemia. An abnormal response in the endometrium may result in focal proliferation of non-secretory cystic glandular hyperplasia resulting in an endometrial polyp. At the menopause, gradual fall in oestrogen activity results in involution of the hyperplasia, but the glands remain cystic—senile cystic endometrium. Atypical hyperplasia differs from simple hyperplasia in that it is focal and shows epithelial atypia. This process predisposes to the development of endometrial adenocarcinoma.

Leiomyoma (fibroid) of myometrium

Approximately one-tenth of all patients in gynaecological practice suffer from fibroids. The tumours show a wide range of presentations. They may be single or multiple and number up to 100. They may be of pinhead size, or be so large as to cause massive distortion of the uterus. Most leiomyomas occupy an intramural position, but some exist as either subserous or submucous polyps, projecting from the peritoneal surface or into the endometrial cavity respectively. Occasionally the tumour will form in the cervical myometrium or extramurally in the broad ligament. Leiomyomas are usually hard and difficult to cut. Their fasciculated pale-grey cut surface has been likened to watered silk. They are prone to degenerative changes, among which necrosis, oedema, haemorrhage, cyst formation and calcification are observable macroscopically. Haemorrhagic necrosis is liable to develop in the pregnant uterus and in those on oral contraceptives (red degeneration). Occasionally the myoma may become completely impregnated with calcium (a 'womb stone'). The histological picture consists of interweaving bundles of smooth muscle fibres in a varying amount of fibrous stroma, which contains a number of medium-sized vascular channels, and frequently undergoes hyaline 'degeneration'. Although the tumour can usually be shelled out from the surrounding myometrium, the line of separation may not be clear cut histologically. The aetiology of these tumours is still obscure. The fact that they are limited to the reproductive era indicates that they are endocrine dependent. Structurally they are similar to the vascular leiomyomas that sometimes develop in the skin. Occasionally leiomyosarcomatous change develops.

Decidual cast

During pregnancy, progestational stimulation of the endometrium results in secretory hyperplasia. The glands become excessively tortuous, the epithelium pale and vacuolated and the nuclei protrude into the lumen. These changes are known as the Arias–Stella phenomenon. The stromal cells acquire abundant cytoplasm to form decidua. If there is a uterine pregnancy, chorionic villi become embedded in this decidua. However, if there is an ectopic (tubal) pregnancy (see p. 196), the endometrial changes occur without chorionic villi. Death of the fetus may be followed by shedding of the endometrium as a decidual cast. Excessive decidua may also accompany prolonged progestogen therapy. If there is no oestrogen priming of the glands, these remain atrophic so that the glands and stroma become 'out of step'. Withdrawal of progestogen may result in a decidual cast being shed.

Endometritis

Chronic inflammation of the endometrium commonly follows abortion; it may be the result of chronic gonococcal infection also affecting the fallopian tubes or it may be due to tuberculosis. Tuberculous granulomas take some weeks to develop so that they are not seen in the postmenstrual or proliferative phase of the menstrual cycle. If tuberculosis is suspected, curettage is best postponed until the premenstrual phase of the cycle. Endometrial tuberculosis is always secondary to tuberculosis elsewhere in the body, particularly in the urinary tract and lungs. Endometritis may occur in older women as a result of endometrial carcinoma.

Carcinoma of the endometrium

Adenocarcinoma of the endometrium is becoming more common. It is commonest in the sixth decade and is particularly associated with obesity, nulliparity, a late menopause and a source of excess oestrogen. Atypical hyperplasia of the endometrium sometimes precedes development of the invasive tumour.

The tumour often projects into the uterine cavity as a papillary mass and irregular or postmenopausal uterine bleeding is a common presenting symptom. At the time of diagnosis, myometrial invasion is often limited to the superficial layers. Tumour may extend into the endocervix and into the submucosal lymphatics in the upper third of the vagina. Most of the tumours are well-differentiated adenocarcinomas. Metastasis to the ovaries is common but the tumour rarely becomes widespread outside the pelvis. Prognosis depends on the stage, but it is generally more favourable than for carcinoma of the cervix.

Endometrial sarcoma

The endometrial stroma may become malignant, producing sheets of undifferentiated cells or there may be differentiation into a variety of mesodermal tissues, including glandular epithelium, to form a mixed mesodermal tumour. Endometrial sarcomas are considerably more malignant than the more common carcinomas and there is often infiltration through the myometrium into the parametrial tissues at the time of clinical presentation.

Adenomyosis

In this condition the myometrium usually shows an asymmetric swelling without clear boundaries, the cut surface of which is coarsely trabeculated; small cystic spaces may be present, which are sometimes blood-stained. Histologically, these cystic spaces are seen to be due to islands of endometrium in the myometrium, the endometrial tubules usually appearing hyperplastic and of non-secretory type. The condition is considered to arise as a result of penetration of the endometrium into the underlying myometrium. Though apparently invasive, it is a benign process. A focal, well-circumscribed form is known as an adenomyoma.

The uterine (fallopian) tubes

Inflammation

Acute and chronic inflammation may result from inflammation elsewhere in the genital tract. Examples are puerperal sepsis, gonorrhoea, and non-specific cervicitis. Tuberculous salpingitis is now a rare disease in Britian. All these inflammatory lesions give an obstructive basis for infertility. The inflammation may lead to accumulation of pus within the lumen (pyosalpinx), or extend to involve the ovary (tubovarian abscess). It may settle to leave a distended tube containing watery fluid (hydrosalpinx).

Ectopic pregnancy

Usually because of the development of previous inflammatory changes in the uterine tube, the progress of a fertilized ovum may become arrested in the tube, leading to an ectopic pregnancy. The pregnancy terminates spontaneously in the early stages, as a consequence of the haemorrhage which results from trophoblastic vascular invasion in this abnormal situation. The lesion is an important cause of an acute abdominal emergency in women. The endometrial changes have been described on p. 194.

Tumours

The uterine tubes are a very uncommon site for primary tumours. They are, however, more frequently involved in extensions of carcinoma from the uterine body or ovaries.

The ovaries

Cysts are prone to develop in the ovaries. For convenience they can be divided into non-neoplastic and neoplastic cysts.

Non-neoplastic cysts

Germinal inclusion cysts

These are usually small, not visible to the naked eye, and are lined by a single layer of cuboidal or columnar cells.

Follicular cysts

These are the commonest cysts to be observed in the ovary, are unilocular, differ from developing follicles in being over 2.5 cm in diameter, and are filled with clear fluid rich in oestrogen. There may be associated non-secretory hyperplasia of the endometrium due to prolonged oestrogen stimulation. Histologically, the cysts are seen to be lined by granulosa and theca interna cells. They may be particularly numerous and prominent in the Stein–Leventhal syndrome in which the combination of amenorrhoea and hirsutism exists.

Corpus luteum cysts

These result when there is an aberration of the normal regression of the corpora lutea. The cyst fluid may be clear or consist of blood.

Endometrial cysts

Ectopic endometrium may be found in the ovary, forming the wall of a cyst. The endometrium is rarely fully developed; the commonest arrangement seen histologically is cuboidal or columnar epithelium lining the cyst with well-developed endometrial stroma, beneath which there may be clusters of siderocytes indicative of previous haemorrhage. The cyst lumen often contains blood. The likely causes of 'chocolate cysts' of ovary are thus haemorrhagic corpus luteum and endometrial cyst.

Parovarian cysts are derived from embryonic Mullerian and Wolffian duct remnants in the hilum of the ovary and lateral end of the fallopian tube. They are simple cysts lined by cubical or flattened epithelium.

Neoplastic cysts

Mucinous cystadenoma

This accounts for 25% of all ovarian tumours, and is the one which produces the biggest forms. The outer surface is smooth and the cut surface is multilocular with thin walls. The cavities are filled with clear mucin. Histologically, the cyst walls are lined by tall columnar epithelium, with basal nuclei and pale cytoplasm because of the contained mucin. Rupture of these cysts, as with similar cystic tumours in the pancreas and appendix, may result in seeding of tumour cells throughout the peritoneal cavity. They continue to produce mucin and give rise to pseudomyxoma (myxoma) peritonei.

Serous cystadenoma

This also accounts for 25% of all ovarian tumours. About 20% are bilateral. The outer surface may be smooth or show fine warty outgrowths. It is commonly unilocular and filled with clear fluid. The inner lining may be smooth or covered with warty ingrowths which are found more frequently than the outgrowths already mentioned. Microscopically, it is seen to be lined by a single layer of flattened epithelium, the warty structures having fibrous cores. Malignant change occurs more frequently than with the mucinous variety.

Dermoid cyst

This accounts for 10% of ovarian tumours. Dermoid cysts are usually smaller than the cystadenomas. They are really teratomas and tissues from all three germ layers may be found. A more accurate name than dermoid cyst is benign cystic teratoma. The lumen is often filled with pale greasy material which may contain abundant hairs. A ridge of tissue projects a little into the lumen at one point on the circumference, in which a tooth or bony structures may be obvious. The histological picture, particularly in this region, shows the lining to be of hair-bearing skin under which may be found a wide variety of tissues consisting of normal-looking cells, but not showing the relationship commonly observed in the normal body. Malignant change in ovarian dermoid tumours is very rare.

Carcinoma of the ovary

Carcinoma of the ovary accounts for approximately 6% of all female deaths from malignant disease. *Primary carcinoma* may be either predominantly cystic or mainly solid, the relative frequency being approximately in the ratio of 4:1. The cystic forms originate in the corresponding cystadenomas and are either serous or mucinous cystadenocarcinomas, the former being much the more common. Features of malignancy in these tumours include solid areas in a cystic tumour, necrosis, infiltration of the capsule and pelvic adhesions. Histologically, there is heaping-up of the lining epithelium with nuclear pleomorphism and mitotic activity. The solid carcinomas are adenocarcinomas which vary in differentiation from case to case. Spread of all forms is usually first to the peritoneum and omentum, so that ascites and adhesions between bowel loops frequently develop. Spread may also take place into the rest of the genital tract, and metastases in the endometrium are common. Pelvic and para-aortic lymph nodes are frequently involved but haematogenous spread is less usual. The five-year survival is approximately 15–20%. Metastases to the pleural cavity may give rise to a malignant effusion. The ovaries are quite frequently the seat of *secondary carcinoma*, the commonest primary sites being the alimentary tract, especially the stomach (Krukenberg tumours), the uterine body and breast. Krukenberg tumours may mimic primary ovarian fibromas, although histologically the mucin-secreting carcinoma cells reveal their true identity. It seems probable that gastric carcinomas invade the ovaries by transperitoneal spread, although in other cases lymphatic and haematogenous spread may be more important.

Functional tumours of the ovary

Some tumours of the ovary produce hormones, mainly oestrogen. The most important of these tumours is derived from, and histologically resembles, the granulosal cells of the developing follicle—the *granulosa cell tumour*. A closely related tumour is the *thecoma*. Both of these tumours are well circumscribed and on section may appear yellow. Granulosa cell tumours often contain cysts or areas of haemorrhage, whereas thecomas more frequently resemble fibromas. Both types of tumour are usually benign in their behaviour, although 30% recur after excision. The effects of the high oestrogen output is to cause endometrial hyperplasia or carcinoma, leiomyomata of the myometrium and cystic hyperplasia of the breast. Masculinizing effects are produced by the *arrhenoblastoma*, a tumour of varying histological pattern but often containing tubular structures and cells resembling the interstitial cells of the testis. About 20% of the tumours recur and metastasize. In addition to these functional tumours, it is now clear that many types of ovarian tumour occasionally may be associated with excess oestrogen production.

Other ovarian tumours

Brenner tumours are benign fibrous tumours which contain islands of squamous epithelium possibly derived from islands of metaplastic surface epithelium commonly found on the fallopian tube and ovary— Walthard's nests. These tumours may occur in the wall of mucinous cystadenomas.

Fibromas are common and are derived from the stroma of the ovarian cortex. The surface epithelium may be invaginated into the fibroma to form an adenofibroma or cystadenofibroma. Some fibromas represent the end-stages of thecomas or Brenner tumours and careful search may be required to identify their true nature.

Dysgerminoma, a rare tumour identical to the seminoma of the testis, arises more commonly in dysgenetic gonads, e.g. Turner's syndrome. It metastasizes to para-aortic lymph nodes and by the bloodstream.

Torsion of the ovary

Torsion of the ovary is usually secondary to an ovarian neoplasm. Those most likely to undergo torsion are heavy, benign tumours on a long pedicle such as dermoid cysts and fibromas. Malignant tumours rarely undergo torsion because of pelvic adhesions. Torsion results in venous occlusion, oedema and infarction of the ovary and attached fallopian tube.

Endometriosis

The presence of ectopic endometrium in the ovary has already been mentioned. It may be found in the uterine tube, on the outside of the uterus, on the pelvic peritoneum, the bowel, the bladder and even the umbilicus, as well as in less frequent sites. Multiple lesions are usual. Macroscopically, the foci of endometriosis are small, usually puckered scars, which contain tar-like blood-stained fluid. Microscopically, the combination of endometrial epithelium and stroma is diagnostic, and tissue reaction to shed blood is usually present. The pathogenesis of this condition is obscure. It may be due to growth of particles of endometrium transported from the uterus through the uterine tube or by metaplastic transformation of tissues having the factor in common that they are derived from primitive coelom. As neither explanation can account for all cases, it is possible that more than one factor is involved in the formation of these lesions.

Tumours of the placenta

Two tumours are derived from the trophoblastic covering of the chorionic villi of the placenta. These are *hydatidiform mole* and *choriocarcinoma*. There is a moderate degree of trophoblastic proliferation in hydatidiform mole; the chorionic villi become hydropic and avascular, resembling small grapes. These are usually benign but may progress to choriocarcinoma. It is interesting that chromosomal analysis of these tumours shows that the cells are of XX type and that both X chromosomes are of paternal origin. In the latter, the trophoblastic proliferation is considerable and it is usually impossible to recognize any villous structure. Choriocarcinoma is a highly malignant and invasive tumour, which often appears haemorrhagic. Both tumours are associated with the secretion of large quantities of *chorionic gonadotrophin* which may give strong-positive pregnancy tests. They also cause the formation of ovarian cysts lined by luteinized theca cells—*theca lutein cysts*.

Pre-eclamptic toxaemia of pregnancy

This disease occurs usually in late pregnancy. It is characterized by hypertension, proteinuria and oedema. In more severe cases the patient has fits, and the condition is then referred to as *eclampsia*. The placenta undergoes premature ageing causing fetal distress. In eclampsia, there is swelling of endothelial cells and thickening of basement membranes in renal glomeruli. The liver may show periportal necrosis which may progress to massive necrosis. The cause of these changes is not completely understood but appears to be related to a placental factor for there is often dramatic improvement following the termination of pregnancy.

21

The Breast

Inflammatory lesions

Breast abscess is usually found in the lactating breast, and is caused by organisms which gain entry through a crack in the nipple. The changes in the breast are those of acute inflammation.

Fat necrosis occurs usually in pendulous breasts following trauma. Fat is released from damaged adipocytes and this sets up a chronic inflammatory reaction in which there are many histiocytes, with some multinucleate forms. The fibrosis which accompanies this process results in a firm mass which can be mistaken for carcinoma.

The changes of fat necrosis are very similar to those seen in some cases of *duct ectasia*. This condition is associated with duct obstruction and dilatation. The secretory contents, rich in lipid, are phagocytosed by macrophages which are identical to the macrophages of fat necrosis. When the duct ruptures, the macrophages spill into the surrounding breast tissue and a chronic inflammatory reaction results. Rarely, the inflammatory cells are almost exclusively plasma cells; the term *plasma cell mastitis* is then used.

True *chronic mastitis* as a result of infection is rare but tuberculosis, blastomycosis or actinomycosis occur. Secondary inflammation associated with proliferative disorders of the breast is much commoner.

Benign proliferative disorders

These include cystic hyperplasia, fibrocystic disease of the breast, and chronic cystic mastitis.

There is a wide range of benign proliferative lesions which present as masses in the female breast after adolescence. Rather than describe each histological appearance as a distinct disease, it is better to group them all under one term, though one particular pattern may predominate in any individual lump.

The commoner changes which are seen are as follows.

1. *Fibrosis*, where the dense interlobular connective tissue extends into the lobules.

2. *Sclerosis*, which is a form of fibrosis where the connective tissue becomes relatively acellular and often distorts glands.

3. *Cysts* of varying size are common (often multiple). They are lined with ductal epithelium and contain turbid fluid. Unopened cysts often have a bluish colour.

4. *Adenosis* is an increase in the number of ductules in the lobules.

5. *Epitheliosis* is a proliferation of the epithelium in a duct, filling and expanding it.

6. *Papillomatosis* is similar to epitheliosis but the proliferating ductal epithelium has a papillary pattern.

7. *Apocrine metaplasia* is a change in the ductal epithelium to tall, columnar, markedly eosinophilic cells resembling those of apocrine sweat glands. A lymphocytic infiltrate frequently accompanies proliferative changes and this gave rise to the term 'cystic mastitis', but this is not a good phrase because the disorder is not primarily inflammatory.

When particular combinations are seen they are sometimes designated fibroadenosis, sclerosing adenosis or cystic change. This has some clinical value, for example sclerosing adenosis can easily be mistaken for carcinoma. Frequently the whole range of changes may be seen in one individual.

The relationship of these changes to the subsequent development of carcinoma is still not precisely known. If the group is taken together, then the increased risk of carcinoma in a woman who has had a benign lump removed is not great. There is some evidence, however, that marked epitheliosis has more sinister significance.

Benign tumours

Fibroadenoma is a common tumour, usually less than 3 cm in diameter. It is a well-circumscribed, firm lump whose cut surface is pearly grey to the naked eye. Histologically, the commonest picture is one of stretched epithelium lining slit-like lumens and being distorted by irregular overgrowth of the characteristically loose fibrous tissue (the intracanalicular form). Less commonly, the tubules are small and circular and are surrounded by whorls of fibrous tissue (the pericanalicular form). The tumours tend to regress with age and may become hyaline, calcified or ossified. An uncommon variant is the *giant intracanalicular fibroadenoma* which tends to occur in older people. These are also called cystosarcoma phyllodes because of the fleshy leaf-like appearance of the cut surface. In behaviour they range from benign to malignant tumours; the name 'cystosarcoma' is misleading for those at the benign end of the scale.

A *duct papilloma* usually occurs as a small solitary tumour in a main duct near the nipple. These papillomas present with bleeding from the nipple rather than as lumps in the breast. They are benign lesions, though occasionally carcinomas can develop from them.

Carcinoma of the breast

Carcinoma of the breast is the commonest cause of death due to cancer in women, accounting for 20% of cancer deaths. About 1 in every 24 females in Britain will eventually die of breast carcinoma, but it is rare in males. It is rare before the age of 25 but increases in frequency each decade thereafter. There is a familial tendency to develop the tumour but it is uncertain whether this is genetic in origin. Abnormal or delayed lactation has long been thought to be associated with the development of breast carcinoma but it is probable that the most important factor is age at first pregnancy. The older the individual at first pregnancy, the greater the risk of breast carcinoma.

The upper and outer quadrant of the breast is the most frequent site affected, the centre and upper inner quadrant next, and the lower segments are the least often involved. The naked-eye appearances vary considerably. The commonest form is a hard (scirrhous) nodule about 1–2 cm across which sends short processes into the adjacent breast tissue. The tumour usually has a concave cut surface which has gritty, yellowish flecks (cutting like an unripe pear). The hardness is due to the dense fibrous tissue formed as a response to the tumour cells. Another type is the *encephaloid* (medullary) growth which is larger and softer; sometimes this is composed of masses of poorly differentiated cells and has a poor prognosis, but occasionally there is a marked lymphoid reaction (*encephaloid carcinoma with lymphoid stroma*) which is presum ably immunological and is a marker of good prognosis. Other naked-eye appearances of the cut surface of tumours are *mucoid* (colloid), due to abundant mucus secretion by tumour cells, *papillary*, where the tumour grows in a papillary pattern, and *comedo*, where parts of the tumour confined within ducts undergo central necrosis giving an appearance reminiscent of comedones. In general, naked-eye appearances, apart from size, are not good indicators of prognosis.

Histologically, breast carcinomas are classified first as *pre-invasive* or *invasive*. There are two forms of pre-invasive carcinoma, *intraduct* and *in-situ lobular*. Intraduct carcinoma shows marked proliferation of cells within the ducts; these show central necrosis, mitotic activity and dysplastic nuclei. When involving the large ducts, it is sometimes associated with *Paget's disease of the nipple*. In this condition the epithelium of the nipple is invaded by large pale-staining cells (Paget's cells) and may present clinically with an eczematoid appearance. Though the nature of these cells is still debated, most people regard them as malignant. In-situ lobular carcinoma has different appearances charac-terized by the ductules filling up with collections of oval, rather even cells. This form is less common and is more easily missed than the intraduct form. The treatment of both forms of pre-invasive carcinoma is controversial. Intraduct carcinoma is frequently localized and many surgeons would treat by local excision alone, though some perform a mastectomy. In-situ lobular is commonly a more widespread change and some believe that further biopsies should be taken before deciding on treatment.

Invasive carcinomas of the breast are usually adenocarcinomas. They have variable appearances but the histological features are not easily translated into clinically useful information. Most of the tumours are of duct pattern and a smaller number are recognizable as being of lobular origin; some contain both patterns. The lobular tumours are more likely to have oestrogen receptors. *Grading* is more difficult than for most tumours, and the widely known scheme which correlates with the prognosis is that of Bloom and Richardson, which involves a time-consuming assessment of pleomorphism, tubule formation and mitotic activity. The only other histological feature that unequivocally indicates a good prognosis is the appearance of the encephaloid tumour with a heavy lymphoid stroma. Staging the tumour in terms of size, skin and muscle involvement, lymph node or distant metastasis gives a better indication of prognosis. Stage I tumours are less than 2 cm in diameter with no evidence of spread. Stage II are between 2 cm and 5 cm in diameter. Stage III tumours show spread to the chest wall or to regional lymph nodes or are greater than 5 cm diameter. Stage IV have distant metastases.

Local spread may involve the skin and make it difficult for it to be moved over the tumour (skin tethering). The skin may become oedematous through lymphatic obstruction (peau d'orange). Nipple retraction is common and the skin may ulcerate. The tumour may also become attached to the chest wall. *Lymphatic spread* occurs early, often involving the axillary and supraclavicular nodes but also spreading to the internal mammary chain. *Blood spread* leads to involvement of lung, liver, brain and bones; the bone involvement may be localized, causing a pathological fracture, or widespread, leading to diminished haemopoiesis. The bony metastases are usually osteolytic but may be osteosclerotic.

Metastases may present years after the primary tumour has been removed and it is realized now that once it has become invasive, breast carcinoma is often a systemic disease, unlikely to be cured by radical surgery directed at the primary tumour. Apart from radiotheraphy and chemotherapy, manipulation of the hormone environment of these tumours may be helpful, for some of them have detectable hormone receptors on their surfaces. How the hormone environment affects the development of a carcinoma is still being investigated.

22

The Thyroid, Parathyroids, Adrenals and Pituitary

The thyroid gland

Goitres

These are enlarged thyroid glands, which may be nodular or diffuse.

The pituitary stimulates the thyroid through the action of thyroid-stimulating hormone (TSH), causing proliferation and increased activity of the thyroid epithelium. In the presence of adequate iodine supplies, this causes an increased output of thyroxine into the blood, which suppresses further pituitary output of TSH. In the absence of adequate iodine supplies, as in mountainous areas or following therapy with goitrogenic substances, the output of thyroxine fails, and the prolonged TSH stimulation of the thyroid causes a *simple goitre*. As expected, the gland is fleshy and cellular with little colloid stored in it. When the demand for thyroxine diminishes or when iodine supplies are restored, the gland undergoes involution with accumulation of large quantities of pale-staining colloid to form a *colloid goitre*. This may be *diffuse* or, with recurrent stimulation and involution, it may become a multinodular goitre. In these nodular goitres, haemorrhage is very likely to occur and results in focal scars or cyst formation. *Toxic goitres* are associated with the increased output of thyroxine either due to an independently functioning nodule or due to the presence in the serum of thyroid-stimulating immunoglobulin. This thyroid overactivity results in thyrotoxicosis (hyperthyroidism). Other causes of goitre are carcinoma and thyroiditis, including Hashimoto's disease. The term 'solitary nodule' refers to a single localized lump in the thyroid, its nature may be that of a reactive nodule, an adenoma, or a carcinoma.

Hyperthyroidism

This disease occurs in two main forms, *exophthalmic goitre* (primary thyrotoxicosis or Graves' disease) and *toxic nodular goitre* (secondary thyrotoxicosis). Graves' disease is associated with the presence in the serum of immunoglobulins directed at the TSH receptors on the follicular cells. The autoantibodies may be detected in a number of different ways, and may be called long-acting thyroid stimulator (LATS) or human thyroid stimulator (HTS). These patients may have other thyroid antibodies in their serum similar to those found in Hashimoto's disease, and some patients with Graves' disease progress to Hashimoto's disease. Graves' disease affects particularly young and middle-aged adults, being much commoner in women. There is exophthalmos and evidence of increased metabolic activity. Some muscle weakness and wasting are common but a fully developed myopathy is rare. Cardiac arrhythmia occurs in older patients. Pretibial myxoedema may develop and is due to the accumulation of mucopolysaccharides in the dermis. The diffusely involved gland is very vascular and firmer than normal. It feels tough on section, the cut surface is fleshy, and colloid is hard to identify. Microscopically, the follicles are hyperplastic, being lined by columnar epithelium thrown up into papillary infoldings. Colloid is scanty and pale staining with peripheral vacuolation where it lies adjacent to follicular cells. Lymphoid follicles with germinal centres are scattered through the gland. Apart from the lymphoid tissue, thought to be a manifestation of autoimmunity, the hyperplastic appearance is not pathognomonic of Graves' disease for it may be due to TSH stimulation and is found in patients treated with carbimazole, which prevents the formation of iodotyrosine and thyroxine, thus stimulating pituitary activity by failure of 'negative feedback'. The histological picture of Graves' disease is usually obscured in the surgically excised gland because preoperative iodine therapy makes the thyroid gland revert in the direction of normal.

Toxic nodules produce excessive quantities of thyroid hormone but it is not associated with high levels of HTS in the serum. Secondary hyperthyroidism occurs in older patients and the overactivity is more likely to be associated with cardiac arrhythmia; exophthalmos is not a feature. Thyrotoxicosis should always be considered in the diagnosis of unexplained cardiac arrhythmia in elderly patients. Radioactive iodine uptake by the gland reveals that it is concentrated in the 'hot nodule'.

Macroscopically and histologically, the nodule shows the features of hyperplasia, but the remainder of the gland shows no clear-cut differences from non-toxic nodular goitre. The reason for a single nodule showing increased function is not yet clear, but the fact that the normal gland shows focal uptake of radioactive iodine may provide part of the explanation.

Thyroiditis

Acute thyroiditis may complicate a local inflammatory reaction such as a carbuncle in the neck or it may be a complication of septicaemia. *Subacute (giant-cell) thyroiditis* (de Quervain's disease) is an inflammatory lesion which presents as a diffuse, tender enlargement of the gland. It is probably of viral origin and cases occur in association with mumps.

Histologically, giant cell—histiocyte granulomas, similar to those found in sarcoid, occur in thyroid follicles and ingest colloid resulting in focal scarring; myxoedema is uncommon. *Hashimoto's disease* (struma lymphomatosa) is an autoimmune form of thyroiditis. It occurs particularly in middle-aged women as a firm, diffuse enlargement of the thyroid gland leading to loss of function and myxoedema. The serum can be shown to contain antibodies to thyroglobulin and various components of thyroid cytoplasm. Some of these patients also have antibodies in their serum which react with gastric parietal cells and may be associated with megaloblastic anaemia due to absence of intrinsic factor (see p. 140). Macroscopically, the gland shows uniform enlargement but remains confined by the capsule. The cut surface is pale. Histologically, there is infiltration by lymphocytes and plasma cells destroying the normal follicular pattern. Colloid is scanty; epithelial cells are aggregated in small foci and show metaplasia to large eosinophilic cells—Askanazy cells. Fibrous tissue gradually replaces the cellular infiltrate and destroyed follicles. *Focal lymphocytic thyroiditis* is found in hyperplastic glands of primary thyrotoxicosis. When this thyroiditis is extensive and associated with the formation of germinal centres, there is a tendency for patients to develop myxoedema. It is, therefore, a feature of some importance in thyroidectomy specimens. It shows many features in common with Hashimoto's disease. *Reidel's thyroiditis* is a rare form of thyroiditis in which there is fibrous replacement of the gland with involvement of surrounding tissues, causing tracheal or oesophageal obstruction. It is usually mistaken clinically for carcinoma. The aetiology of the disease is not known. In spite of extensive destruction of the gland, myxoedema is seen in only a minority of cases.

Hypothyroidism

In children this may be the result of congenital absence of the thyroid gland or failure of one of the enzyme systems in the gland necessary for the formation of thyroxine (dyshormonogenetic goitre). It may be due to iodine deficiency during intrauterine life. In adults Hashimoto's disease is one of the most important causes of hypothyroidism. Primary atrophy (chronic atrophic thyroiditis) may develop in adult life, the histological picture being that of atrophy with fibrous replacement of follicles, but lymphocytic infiltration is usually slight. Antithyroid drugs, thyroidectomy, irradiation and pituitary failure may all cause loss of thyroid function. The result is the clinical picture of *cretinism* in infants and *myxoedema* in adults. A cretin shows failure of mental and physical development. The skin is cold, dry and puffy; the tongue is large and protudes. Myxoedema in adults may be inapparent until it has reached an advanced stage. The puffiness of the skin is caused by infiltration of the dermis by mucopolysaccharides. The skin is cold, the hair brittle, scanty and dry. There is hoarseness due to swelling of the vocal cords.

Hyperlipidaemia leads to coronary ischaemia but this may be less obvious clinically in untreated cases due to bradycardia and low cardiac output. Impairment of mental function may result in psychoses or coma.

Tumours

Adenoma

The distinction between adenoma and the nodules of a nodular goitre is not clear. The term 'adenoma' is usually reserved for a nodule which is well circumscribed, surrounded by a fibrous capsule, compressing the adjacent thyroid tissue and having a histological pattern different from the rest of the gland. An adenoma is usually fleshy and histologically the follicles may resemble immature (fetal adenoma) or mature (follicular adenoma) thyroid. These tumours are prone to haemorrhage and cystic degeneration. Haemorrhage into a retrosternal adenoma may cause sudden and severe obstruction of the thoracic inlet. Very few adenomas have been shown to undergo malignant change.

Carcinoma

This is a relatively rare cause of death from malignant disease but it is important in that it often affects young adults and the metastases may be suitable for treatment with radioactive iodine. Irradiation of the neck or mediastinum in childhood increases the risk of developing carcinoma but there is usually a latent period of 10 years or more before the tumour develops. The likelihood of radio-iodine therapy causing carcinoma in an adult is very small. Four main types are described. (1) *Papillary carcinoma* affects a younger age group than the other patterns of carcinoma. The primary tumour is often very small but it metastasizes early to cervical lymph nodes. Because the primary tumour may be undetectable clinically, these metastases have been erroneously called 'lateral aberrant thyroid'. In spite of early lymph node metastases, these tumours often remain confined to the neck and have a relatively good prognosis. (2) *Follicular carcinoma* resembles, sometimes very closely, normal thyroid gland. It shows a greater tendency to spread by way of the bloodstream, especially to the lungs and bones. It is this pattern of tumour which is best suited to radio-iodine therapy. During initial thyroidectomy, lymph node metastases in the neck are also surgically removed. Distant metastases may then be susceptible to ^{131}I therapy. (3) *Medullary carcinoma* arises from parafollicular (C) cells and does not produce colloid. It occurs over a wide age range and has a variable prognosis. It shows accumulation of amyloid. Some of these tumours are familial and there may be associated lesions such as mucocutaneous polyps and adrenal phaeochromocytoma. (4) *Anaplastic carcinoma* may either be of small cell or giant cell pattern. These are rapidly growing tumours which metastasize readily by lymphatics and bloodstream. Most do not concentrate iodine and so are not amenable to radio-iodine therapy. The prognosis is poor. Small cell carcinoma may be confused with primary malignant lymphoma of the thyroid.

The parathyroid glands

The parathyroid glands impinge on the clinical scene as a result of either under-production or over-production of parathormone. The commonest cause of underactivity leading to tetany is ablation, usually as a complication of thyroidectomy. Overactivity can arise spontaneously, or secondarily to the usual stimulus for parathormone production, i.e. a low serum calcium. In clinical practice, the latter is most commonly due to impaired calcium absorption of chronic renal disease, and leads to hyperplasia of all the glands. Spontaneous or primary overactivity is most commonly a consequence of a functioning adenoma in one of the glands or, rarely, it is due to primary hyperplasia or carcinoma. An independently functioning adenoma can occasionally develop in secondary hyperplasia (tertiary hyperparathyroidism). Adenomas vary in size, averaging about 300 mg (normal total weight of four parathyroids <120 mg) and are usually of orange-brown colour. Histologically they consist predominantly of dark chief cells, although some tumours are mainly oxyphil cells. A rim of normal parathyroid is compressed around the tumour. Occasionally a parathyroid adenoma may be associated with similar tumours of pancreatic islets and pituitary (multiple endocrine adenomatosis type I—Wermer's syndrome). In hyperplasia the whole gland is involved, due mainly to chief cell hyperplasia, and the cytoplasm of these cells may be vacuolated or 'water-clear'. The commonest effect of primary parathyroid overactivity is to cause mobilization of calcium from the bones and increased excretion of calcium and phosphate by the kidneys. The mobilization of calcium causes hypercalcaemia and metastatic calcification in organs such as the kidneys, with the formation of renal calculi. The bones become diffusely decalcified. Histologically, seams of uncalcified bone matrix (osteoid) may be found covering the bone trabeculae. There may be focal destruction of bone due to osteoclast activity. Haemorrhage and cyst formation occur with fibrous replacement of the destroyed bone. Many osteoclasts are found in the lesions. These changes produce the 'brown tumours' of osteitis fibrosa cystica (von Recklinghausen's disease of bone) which may be misdiagnosed as giant cell tumours of bone (osteoclastoma).

The adrenal glands

It is convenient to consider the adrenal as consisting of two independent endocrine glands, the cortex and the medulla. The cortex is divided into three zones: an outer zona glomerulosa, an intermediate zona fasciculata and an inner zona reticularis. These zones react differently in various pathological states. Diseases of the cortex may result in either increased or decreased function.

Decreased cortical activity

Acute cortical insufficiency may result from massive bilateral adrenal haemorrhage causing destruction of the whole cortex. This is found as a complication of severe infection, particularly meningococcal septicaemia (Waterhouse–Friderichsen syndrome). There is often evidence of intravascular thrombosis similar to that which may be produced in the generalized Shwartzman phenomenon.

Chronic cortical insufficiency leads to the development of *Addison's disease* in which there is skin pigmentation, wasting, weakness and hypotension; there may also be anorexia, nausea and vomiting. There is loss of sodium in the urine leading to hyponatraemia and uraemia. Tuberculosis was the commonest cause of chronic cortical insufficiency in the past but, with the reduction in the number of cases of tuberculosis, this has become less important, and the condition is now more commonly due to primary atrophy. The latter is an autoimmune disease in which there is lymphocytic infiltration of the cortex, with destruction of cortical cells and fibrous replacement. Some cases of primary atrophy also have antibodies to thyroid and gastric parietal cells. Secondary carcinoma and amyloidosis are rare causes of Addison's disease. Hypopituitarism may lead to secondary atrophy of the adrenal cortex. Skin pigmentation is not a feature of the latter due to the low output of melanophore-stimulating hormone (MSH) by the pituitary.

Increased cortical activity

Increased cortical activity may result in excessive production of one or more of the three main hormone groups, the C21 steroids (cortisol, corticosterone, and aldosterone), the C19 steroids (androgens) and the C18 steroids (oestrogens). The associated structural changes may be bilateral hyperplasia, adenoma or carcinoma.

Congenital adrenal hyperplasia (adrenogenital syndrome) is a group of disorders in which impaired cortisol synthesis results in raised ACTH levels and subsequent abnormalities of androgen, and sometimes mineralocorticoid, production. The commonest form is 21-hydroxylase deficiency which gives impaired cortisol and aldosterone deficiency with virilism resulting from excess androgen production. The clear cells of the zona fasciculata become replaced by compact cells similar to those of the zona reticularis.

Cushing's syndrome is characterized by obesity (mainly of the trunk), plethora, skin striae, hypertension, osteoporosis and diabetes mellitus. It may be due to predominant secretion of C21 steroids or there may be a mixture of C21 and C19 steroids in which case virilism will also be present. Most adult cases are due to bilateral cortical hyperplasia caused by overstimulation by the pituitary (Cushing's disease). Some cases show small basophil adenomas of the pituitary and in a few there may be chromophobe pituitary adenomas. In children, and less commonly in adults, adenoma or carcinoma of the adrenal cortex may be the primary pathology. In these cases there is independent function by the tumour producing large quantities of cortisol, which suppresses ACTH production by the pituitary causing atrophy of the contralateral adrenal cortex. Bilateral hyperplasia of the cortex and Cushing's syndrome may also be caused by corticotrophin produced by bronchial oat cell carcinoma.

Primary aldosteronism (Conn's syndrome) is due to an adenoma or hyperplasia of the zona glomerulosa of the adrenal cortex. The adenomata are golden yellow and rarely exceed 1 cm in diameter. Aldosterone causes sodium retention and potassium wastage in the urine. There is hypertension and profound weakness due to hypokalaemia. Aldosterone secretion is controlled mainly by the renin–angiotensin system; the zona glomerulosa is stimulated to produce aldosterone by angiotensin which is formed by the action of renin on angiotensinogen in blood. Renin is found in the juxtaglomerular cells of the afferent arteriole in renal glomeruli. Abnormalities of renin production may therefore cause secondary hyperplasia of the adrenal zona glomerulosa (secondary aldosteronism).

Overproduction of oestrogen by the adrenal is rare and usually associated with cortical carcinoma. It causes precocious puberty in girls and feminization in men.

Cortical adenoma is a common finding at post-mortem and in most cases appears to be without clinical hormonal effect. These adenomas are usually less than 1 cm in diameter and golden-yellow in colour. Histologically, they are composed of pale cells resembling those found in the zona fasciculata.

Cortical carcinoma is usually much larger than adenoma. It may show pleomorphism and mitotic activity, but often these tumours mimic adenomas in their histological appearance. Invasion, necrosis and haemorrhage are all sinister features. They metastasize by the blood-stream to the lungs and the prognosis is poor.

Reduced medullary activity

No syndrome can be attributed to diminished medullary function. This is not surprising, for removal of both adrenals necessitates supplements of cortical steroids only.

Increased medullary activity

Phaeochromocytoma

Increased medullary activity is produced pathologically most frequently by a tumour of the noradrenaline- and adrenaline-secreting cells, the phaeochromocytoma. This is usually benign, its average diameter being approx. 4 cm, though occasionally it may be much larger. Its cut surface may be cystic and haemorrhagic, and usually turns strikingly dark brown on exposure to air. The cells have an affinity for chrome salts (chromaffin). Histologically, the tumour shows the presence of large cells, with abundant pink granular cytoplasm loosely arranged round a sinusoidal network. The tumour is one of the less common known causes of hypertension but is nevertheless an important one because its removal leads to cure in early cases. It may be associated with medullary carcinoma of the thyroid (Sipple's syndrome, multiple endocrine adenomatosis type II) or neurofibromatosis. Rarely, phaeochromocytoma may arise in the sympathetic chain outside the adrenal.

Non-functioning tumours

These are usually taken to include neuroblastoma and ganglioneuroma, although occasionally these may be associated with hypertension. Neuroblastoma is a tumour of infancy and childhood, being uncommon above the age of seven. It is frequently haemorrhagic and consists of immature neural tissue arranged in sheets or rosettes. Some neuroblastomas mature to ganglioneuromas; this is more likely with congenital tumours. Most are highly malignant and metastasize by the bloodstream to bone and liver, by lymphatics to regional lymph nodes, and by direct invasion of surrounding structures. Ganglioneuromas occur more frequently in the sympathetic chain but 10% occur in the adrenal medulla. They are firm, fibrous tumours, usually encapsulated. Histologically, they consist of bundles of fibrous tissue with foci of mature ganglion cells. These tumours are benign although transitional forms to neuroblastoma may be found.

Secondary carcinoma

The adrenal is one of the commonest sites for metastatic carcinoma, especially from primary carcinoma in the bronchus. In spite of massive replacement of the gland, it rarely gives symptoms of adrenal insufficiency.

Pituitary

The pituitary is best regarded as two endocrine glands. The anterior lobe (adenohypophysis), which is formed from Rathke's pouch, is composed of cells which, on the basis of the staining characteristics of their cytoplasm in a haematoxylin and eosin stain, are described as basophil (10%), acidophil (40%) or chromophobe cells (50%). These staining characteristics are given by the granules of secretion contained in the cytoplasm. Chromophobes are cells which do not contain enough secretion for their character to be detected. More sensitive techniques using labelled antibodies to the hormones reveal the nature of the cells more precisely.

Basophils and their related chromophobes are responsible for secreting adrenocorticotrophic hormone (ACTH), follicle-stimulating hormone (FSH), luteinizing hormone (LH), and thyroid-stimulating hormone (TSH or thyrotropic hormone). Acidophils and related chromophobes produce growth hormone and prolactin. The secretions of the adenohypophysis are regulated mainly by releasing factors produced in the hypothalamus which reach the anterior pituitary via the special portal blood supply. The posterior pituitary (neurohypophysis) is the source of antidiuretic hormone (ADH) and oxytocin. These hormones are formed in the hypothalamus and pass along nerves, to be released in the posterior pituitary.

Hypopituitarism

This may be idiopathic or result from trauma, pressure from tumours within or adjacent to the pituitary, and interference with the blood supply. In children, panhypopituitarism may either produce *Fröhlich's syndrome*—obesity, mental retardation and genital hypoplasia—or the *Lorain–Levi syndrome*—symmetric dwarfism and genital hypoplasia. In adults, hypopituitarism is most often associated with post-partum infarction of the pituitary as a result of shock due to haemorrhage—*Sheehan's syndrome*. This may become manifest by a failure of lactation and subsequently of continued amenorrhoea. There is loss of pubic axillary hair and the skin is thin and dry. Lack of growth hormone causes atrophy of organs and lack of trophic hormones causes failure of other endocrine glands, particularly the thyroid and later the adrenal cortex.

Failure of the neurohypophysis results in *diabetes insipidus* due to lack of ADH. This causes polyuria and polydipsia.

Hyperpituitarism

Acromegaly is due to an acidophil adenoma producing excess growth hormone. There is enlargement of the jaw, hands and feet, coarsening of the skin, enlargement of other organs such as liver, kidneys and heart, and diabetes mellitus. Before fusion of epiphyses excessive secretion of growth hormone results in *gigantism*.

Cushing's syndrome may be associated with a small basophil adenoma of the pituitary; less commonly, a chromophobe adenoma may be the cause. These tumours cause excessive secretion of ACTH resulting in bilateral cortical hyperplasia of the adrenal.

Inappropriate secretion of antidiuretic hormone may be due to tumours outside the neurohypophysis, notably oat cell carcinoma of the bronchus.

Tumours

Tumours of the anterior pituitary are adenomas derived from chromophobe, acidophil or basophil cells. Chromophobe tumours are often non-functional; by compression of surrounding tissue they may cause hypopituitarism. The largest adenomas are chromophobe; basophil adenomas are usually microscopic in size. *Rathke's pouch cysts* occur between the anterior and posterior parts of the pituitary causing pressure effects on these structures. The cysts are lined by ciliated epithelium.

Craniopharyngiomas are derived from remnants of Rathke's pouch. They may be cystic or solid and composed of squamous epithelium, or they may resemble adamantinoma of the jaw. They are slow growing, locally malignant tumours, found most often above the pituitary.

Gliomas may arise in the neurohypophysis but are rare. *Meningiomas* may occur in the vicinity of the pituitary fossa and mimic pituitary tumours.

Secondary carcinoma in the pituitary was seen commonly in patients undergoing hypophysectomy for advanced breast carcinoma. There may be direct infiltration of the pituitary from nasopharyngeal carcinomas.

23

The Haemopoietic and Allied Systems

The haemopoietic tissue, the lymphoid system and the mononuclear phagocyte system are closely related, both in their embryological origin and in their pathology. Disease processes can affect one element in these systems or several can be involved, especially when a neoplasm occurs. The haemopoietic tissue in the adult is usually found in the bone marrow but in pathological states it can occur elsewhere, particularly in the liver and spleen. The lymphocytes and their derivatives are found almost everywhere in the body but are particularly concentrated in lymph nodes, spleen, gut, bone marrow and, in the child, in the thymus. The macrophages of the mononuclear phagocyte system are found in most tissue but they are particularly prominent in the sinusoids of spleen, liver and lymph nodes.

The anaemias

Anaemia is the state in which the circulating red cell mass is significantly less than normal and the oxygen-carrying capacity of the blood is correspondingly reduced. It is diagnosed by finding a lowered haemoglobin level in the blood. Red cells are formed from their nucleated precursors, the normoblasts, in the bone marrow. They enter the bloodstream when they are mature and stay there on average for 120 days. The ageing cells are then taken up by the cells of the mononuclear phagocyte system (mainly in the spleen) and broken down. The catabolism of haemoglobin yields globin (which is re-utilized), haemosiderin (containing iron which is re-utilized), and bilirubin which is excreted through the liver. In characterizing an anaemia, two measurements are particularly useful. One is the size of the cells (mean corpuscular volume, MCV) which can be microcytic, normocytic or macrocytic. The other is the content of haemoglobin in the cells (the mean corpuscular haemoglobin concentration, MCHC) which can be hypochromic, normochromic or hyperchromic. Anaemia may be due to (1) blood loss, (2) decreased red cell production, or (3) haemolysis.

1. *Blood loss* may be acute or chronic. After an acute large bleed there may be shock, but initially the haemoglobin level will not be low, until the plasma volume has been restored when the dilution effect will result

in a normochromic normocytic anaemia. Chronic loss of blood leads to an iron deficiency anaemia which is microcytic and hypochromic.

2. *Decreased red cell production* may result from many factors but gives rise to three main patterns of anaemia.

a. Microcytic hypochromic anaemias are most commonly due to *iron deficiency* resulting either from dietary deficiency or from chronic blood loss.

Sideroblastic anaemias give a similar peripheral blood picture but in the bone marrow there are abnormal normoblasts with a ring of iron-containing granules around the nucleus—the so-called ring sideroblasts. In these disorders there is a defect in the synthesis of haem, and the normoblasts accumulate iron which they cannot use properly. The *thalassaemias* are hereditary anaemias in which there is a defect in synthesis of the subunits of haem. One or more of the subunits is manufactured in inadequate quantities, though it is qualitatively normal.

b. Macrocytic anaemias are often accompanied by megaloblastic erythropoiesis. The appearance of megaloblasts (large, abnormal normoblasts) in the bone marrow is usually due to a deficiency of a vital nutrient, either vitamin B_{12} or folic acid. Vitamin B_{12} deficiency is seen in pernicious anaemia when it is accompanied by gastric atrophy. Folic-acid deficiency may be due to a deficient diet, but is most often seen in pregnancy or in patients with malabsorption.

c. Normochromic normocytic anaemias may be due to bone marrow disease or may accompany chronic systemic disorders. Examples of primary bone marrow disorders are aplastic anaemia, leukaemia, lymphoma and myelofibrosis. Systemic disorders include uraemia, chronic liver disease, and many forms of chronic inflammation.

3. *Haemolytic anaemias* are those in which red cells have a shorter life span than normal. They can be divided into (i) those where the red cells are structurally defective, and (ii) those where antibodies to the red cells are circulating in the blood. The best-known examples of the first group are hereditary spherocytosis and sickle cell anaemia. Rhesus haemolytic disease of the newborn and autoimmune haemolytic anaemia are examples of the second group.

4. *Mixed pictures* may be seen in some chronic diseases where bleeding, marrow suppression, deficiency of vital elements and haemolysis can all contribute.

Pathological features of anaemia

The bone marrow

This may be studied by way of biopsy during life, such as an iliac trephine or rib biopsy, or at autopsy, when the sternum, vertebral column and femur are usually examined. The information obtained both macroscopically and microscopically is limited; and it should also be remembered that red marrow is normally more extensive in children than adults. In aplastic anaemia the red marrow, usually to be seen in the adult head of the femur at autopsy, is replaced by fat, and the vertebrae and sternum appear a yellowish pink. In all other primary anaemias the red marrow is more abundant than normal. This can only be detected with the naked eye in the adult at autopsy by observing that the red marrow is to be seen farther down the shaft of the femur than normal. Histologically, the balance between haemopoietic and fat cells gives an indication of red cell activity. The red cell precursors can usually be distinguished from white cell precursors in the marrow, but the finer abnormalities of the former, which are of diagnostic value, such as the change to megaloblasts in pernicious anaemia, are best diagnosed in fresh haematologically stained films. The lesions bringing about secondary anaemias such as metastatic carcinoma and leukaemia have, of course, the characteristic pathological features of those diseases.

Iron stores

If red cell breakdown is in excess of red cell formation, there will be a build-up of iron stores in the body. This most commonly occurs in haemolytic and pernicious anaemias. If the prussian blue reaction is carried out at post-mortem on slices of liver and spleen, where the cells of the reticuloendothelial system are abundant, a strongly positive reaction will be obtained in these diseases. Inability to find iron histologically anywhere in the reticuloendothelial tissues supports a diagnosis of iron deficiency, but this examination is rarely necessary for diagnosis.

The tissues

Anaemia is a cause of tissue anoxia. When death takes place after a severe acute anaemia, such as following a massive haemorrhage, all organs will look very pale at autopsy. If the anaemia is more chronic, such as in iron deficiency or pernicious anaemia, degenerative changes may be observed in the tissue cells, the most common of which is fatty change, most easily observed macroscopically in the liver and myocardium (see p. 6).

The myeloproliferative disorders

This term was introduced to link together a number of proliferative disorders of the granulocyte (myeloid) series, erythroid series and megakaryocytes. The reason for linking them together is that there is overlap in their manifestations and often transition of one type to another. The term covers polycythaemia rubra vera, myelofibrosis, essential haemorrhagic thrombocythaemia, acute and chronic granulocytic leukaemia, erythroleukaemia and a few rarer disorders.

Polycythaemia rubra vera

This shows a proliferation of red cell precursors and megakaryocytes. It leads to an increased red cell mass and an expanded circulation, together with increased numbers of platelets and granulocytes. The clinical manifestations result from its effects on the circulation. Dyspnoea on exertion, ankle oedema and angina are frequent complaints, but the most serious complications are thrombosis, haemorrhage and the development of leukaemia—all of which often result in death. It is important to distinguish this disorder from pure red cell increase (erythrocytosis) which is most commonly secondary to some other disease causing anoxia.

Myelofibrosis

This is a slowly progressive disease characterized by anaemia, a raised white cell count, splenomegaly and a failure to aspirate marrow on diagnostic puncture (the 'dry tap'). The histological picture of a fibrotic marrow is characteristic, showing abnormal haemopoiesis, increased fibrosis with fibroblasts and other mononuclear cells. The spleen, liver and lymph nodes show foci of extramedullary haemopoiesis. Many of the features are similar to those of chronic myeloid leukaemia and there may be difficulty in distinguishing the two. The Philadelphia chromosome is found only rarely in myelofibrosis.

Essential haemorrhagic thrombocythaemia

This is a rare disease leading to the appearance in the blood of greatly increased numbers of platelets, which may function abnormally. Both haemorrhages and thromboses occur as complications.

The leukaemias

These are neoplasms derived from any of the haemopoietic cell lines, their effects being most prominent on the bloodstream. They contrast with the malignant lymphomas which are solid tumours of lymphoid (and mononuclear phagocyte) tissue. They account for about 3% of all cancer deaths, are increasing in frequency and may occur at all ages. Most cases occur as one of three fairly well-defined forms: acute leukaemia, chronic myeloid leukaemia, and chronic lymphocytic leukaemia. Myelomonocytic leukaemia is a variant of myeloid leukaemia. Erythroleukaemia (diGuglielmo's disease) is rare.

The cause of leukaemia is not known but ionizing radiation and exposure to some chemicals, such as benzene, are associated with an increased incidence. Some congenital disorders, notably Down's syndrome, are also predisposing factors. In animals, virus infections produce leukaemia but a viral aetiology has still to be proved in man although recent evidence has linked a retrovirus with a T lymphocyte leukaemia in some patients from the Caribbean and Japan.

Acute leukaemia

This form is showing the most striking increase. It is one of the commonest malignant diseases in childhood, but another peak of increasing incidence occurs in old age. It may complicate chronic myeloid leukaemia ('myeloblastic transformation'). Its onset is sudden and its progress, untreated, is rapid. The bone marrow becomes packed with primitive white cells (leucoblasts), so that macroscopically the red marrow takes on a purplish hue. The replacement of fatty marrow by red marrow may not, however, be extensive, presumably because of the short duration of disease before death. The leucoblasts also appear in the blood, though in variable numbers. Evidence of leukaemic proliferation in extramedullary sites may be present, but is uncommonly extensive. The spleen may be slightly enlarged and some of the lymph nodes may be swollen and of purplish colour. Acute leukaemia causes rapid deterioration of the patient, mainly because of its effect on haemopoiesis. Rapidly progressive anaemia is common, and is reflected in the pallor of the viscera observed at autopsy. Purpura is also frequently observed, as a result of the thrombocytopenia which develops. The ulceration of mucous membranes, especially within the mouth, is probably in part due to the severe reduction of neutrophil polymorphs which occurs in this disease (neutropenia, agranulocytosis). There are two major cytological types with similar clinical features but very different responses to treatment. They are distinguished as acute lymphoblastic leukaemia and acute myeloblastic leukaemia. The former responds well to aggressive chemotherapy, especially in childhood, and many cases go into long-term remission. Acute myeloblastic leukaemia is much more resistant to treatment.

Chronic myeloid leukaemia

This disease is nearly as frequent as acute leukaemia and is most common in middle age. It consists of an uncontrolled proliferation of the cells of the granular series, with the result that large numbers of cells of all degrees of maturation appear in the bloodstream. The Philadelphia chromosome is present in the leukaemic cells in 95% of cases. There is usually a great expansion of active marrow, so that at autopsy the whole shaft of the femur will be seen to contain this purplish tissue.

Extramedullary proliferation of cells is usually striking, and may occur in many situations, but tends to be particularly evident in the spleen, which is usually greatly enlarged. The cut surface is swollen, soft and without architectural detail; infarcts and perisplenitis are common. The onset of the disease is more insidious than in acute leukaemia, and the interference with normal haemopoiesis less dramatic. The survival time after diagnosis is on average about three years.

Chronic lymphocytic leukaemia

This is a little less common than the other two variants, and tends to occur in the older age groups. It consists of an uncontrolled proliferation of lymphoid tissue with the result that large numbers of small lymphocytes are produced at these sites, and appear in the blood. It is not surprising that swelling of lymph nodes is a common and dominant feature, but other tissues containing lymphoid follicles also frequently enlarge. The bone marrow is usually packed with lymphocytes by the time the patient is first seen, and the spleen and liver are moderately enlarged. The natural history and the effects on normal haemopoiesis are similar to those of chronic myeloid leukaemia, though a higher proportion run a relatively benign course. There is often some degree of haemolytic anaemia in these cases.

Multiple myeloma

This is a disease caused by the neoplastic proliferation of plasma cells derived from one parent cell (monoclonal). Since each plasma cell is responsible for the production of a specific immunoglobulin, it follows that all plasma cells derived from one parent cell will produce the same type of immunoglobulin. The neoplastic proliferation of these cells suppresses normal plasma cells with the result that other immunoglobulins in the serum are diminished or lost. The sharp band seen on electrophoresis of serum proteins from patients with multiple myeloma indicates a monoclonal immunoglobulin. The abnormal plasma cells synthesize excess light chains (see p. 27) which are excreted in the urine as Bence Jones protein. Multiple myeloma is a disease which is usually confined to the bone marrow. There is diffuse plasma cell infiltration of the marrow; foci of soft deep-red tumour destroy the bone and commonly cause pathological fractures. Histologically, the tumour cells may be mature or primitive plasma cells. The kidney may be severely damaged, either because of accumulation of protein in tubules with obstruction to urine flow or because of massive deposition of amyloid in glomeruli, blood vessels and around tubules. The serum calcium is usually raised. Anaemia is common, but myeloma cells are rarely to be found in the blood. There is evidence that plasma cell proliferation takes

10 to 15 years before it causes clinical disease, but following the onset of symptoms, death usually results within two years.

The malignant lymphomas

These neoplasms produce tumour masses particularly in lymph nodes but also in almost any organ in which lymphocytes are found. They differ from leukaemias in that tumour cells are not prominent in the bloodstream. They differ from most other malignant tumours in having more pronounced systemic effects and often being multicentric at an early stage. They account for about 3% of all deaths from malignancy.

The swollen lymph nodes are usually pale grey-brown, homogeneous and moist on section. If other viscera are involved, the tumour will show similar appearances. Histologically, the common change shown by all forms of lymphoma is the obliteration of the normal lymph node architecture by the proliferation of tumour cells.

There is a wide spectrum of prognosis and response to treatment, so the lymphomas have to be classified into subgroups. This has led to some confusion, for many new classifications have been introduced and there is disagreement amongst experts as to the best way of subdividing them. The division into Hodgkin's and non-Hodgkin's lymphomas is universal. Non-Hodgkin's lymphomas used to be divided into lymphosarcoma, composed of cells recognizable as lymphocytes, and reticulum cell sarcoma, composed of larger cells with bigger nuclei and more cytoplasm. These two types of tumour (the latter having the worse prognosis) were identified before much was known about the physiology of the lymphocyte. As knowledge advanced, so the idea of a reticulum cell retreated and finally disappeared when no one could say what it was. It is now recognized that most of these larger cells are lymphocyte derivatives, though a few of them are true histiocytes (cells of the mononuclear phagocyte system).

Hodgkin's disease

This is the commonest variant, accounting for about half the cases. It is most common between the ages of 20 and 40 but may occur at any age, usually presenting with lymphadenopathy, but sometimes with fever, night sweats, weight loss and pruritus. The enlarged lymph nodes tend to remain discrete and rubbery and the spleen cut surface often appears blotchy, being a pale and dark-brown colour, traditionally likened to 'hard-bake' toffee (i.e. toffee with nuts). Hodgkin's tissue shows a mixture of cells including lymphocytes, larger mononuclear cells and sometimes obvious inflammatory cells including eosinophils. Though the cell of origin of this tumour is still not known, the characteristic cell is binucleate with the nuclei lying side by side in mirror-image form and containing prominent nucleoli; this is the Reed–Sternberg giant cell. The histological picture varies from case to case; three types are recognized depending on the proportion of lymphocytes. These are *lymphocyte predominant, mixed cellularity,* and *lymphocyte depleted.* A fourth type is distinguished by the formation of nodules and fibrosis—*nodular sclerosing Hodgkin's disease.* A better prognosis is associated with lymphocyte predominance and the nodular sclerosing type. Another major determinant of prognosis is the stage of the disease at the time of diagnosis. This is so important in directing treatment that a staging laparotomy is often carried out. Stage I disease involves one group of nodes, Stage II disease is two or more groups above *or* below the diaphragm. Stage III is disease above *and* below the diaphragm. Splenic or extranodal involvement also puts a case into this stage. Stage IV includes disseminated extranodal organ involvement. Limited disease is associated with a better prognosis.

Non-Hodgkin's lymphomas

These usually present with painless lymphadenopathy, sometimes with splenomegaly. Occasionally primary involvement of a major organ, such as the stomach, occurs. A simple classification is based on two observations: one is the architecture of the tumour and the other includes the features of the tumour cells themselves. A nodular architecture (*nodular lymphoma*) is associated with a better prognosis than one composed of diffuse sheets of tumour cells (*diffuse lymphoma*). A tumour composed of small, round lymphocytes (*well-differentiated lymphocytic lymphoma*) has a better prognosis than one composed of poorly differentiated cells which are not easy to recognize as lymphocytes (*poorly differentiated lymphocytic lymphoma* or *lymphoblastic lymphoma*). All the nodular non-Hodgkin's lymphomas and most of the diffuse lymphomas are of B lymphocyte cell type. Some of the diffuse lymphomas are T lymphocyte type and some are true histiocytes, but these are very rare. *Burkitt's lymphoma* is a diffuse lymphoma of B cells occurring particularly in children in Africa, usually with extranodal involvement, typically in the bones of the jaw.

The better prognosis groups, like the better prognosis groups of Hodgkin's disease, are now curable with modern methods of chemotherapy and radiotherapy. The poor prognosis groups are modified by treatment but are not often cured. A degree of immunosuppression is part of the natural history of many malignant lymphomas and this is made worse by treatment methods. It is therefore not surprising to find opportunistic infections in these patients and infection is frequently the cause of death.

Thymus

The relationship of the thymus to immunity has already been indicated (see p. 215). Thymic *hypoplasia* is found in children of both sexes. It may be associated with failure of T lymphocytes (DiGeorge syndrome) or it may be apparently inherited as a recessive gene combined with agammaglobulinaemia and failure of development of lymphoid tissues— a mixed T and B lymphocyte failure (Swiss type agammaglobulinaemia). Thymic *hyperplasia* is found in a variety of conditions, some of which are accepted as being autoimmune diseases. They include Graves' disease, primary atrophy of the adrenal, myasthenia gravis and disseminated lupus erythematosus.

Thymomas may be benign or malignant, but even the latter are only locally infiltrative and rarely metastasize. They may consist mainly of lymphoid cells or of the epithelial component, but it is the latter which is the neoplastic tissue in the tumours. About 40% of patients with a thymoma show features of myasthenia gravis (see p. 235). Some of these patients have improvement in their myasthenia following excision of the tumour. Other cases of thymoma are associated with haemopoietic abnormality, particularly red cell aplasia.

It may be impossible to distinguish between malignant lymphoma or secondary carcinoma in the anterior mediastinum and thymoma. Some cases of Cushing's syndrome reported as being due to thymoma are probably due to metastatic oat cell carcinoma of lung which has a well-recognized association with this syndrome.

Teratoma may occur in the anterior mediastinum as may tumours identical to testicular seminomas (germinoma).

Haemorrhagic disorders

These may be due to defects of the wall of small vessels, changes in platelets, or abnormalities of the plasma factors in the coagulation cascade. Platelet and vessel wall changes tend to be associated with purpura, which is bleeding from small vessels visible on skin or other surfaces; pin-point purpuric spots are called petechiae, larger bleeds are seen as eccymoses (bruises). The most serious small vessel bleeds are those which occur in the brain where they may enlarge and cause death. Coagulation disorders are more often associated with bleeds from larger vessels, for example into joints and soft tissue. The unravelling of the cause of a bleeding disorder is one of the major functions of a haematology laboratory. Classical examples of vessel wall abnormalities are scurvy (vitamin C deficiency, which leads to vessel wall defects due to defective collagen) and the rare hereditary haemorrhagic telangiectasia, where there is fragility of abnormally dilated capillaries. Infections, hypersensitivity reactions and Cushing's syndrome may all produce defects, but perhaps the commonest is senile purpura, most often seen on the extensor surfaces of the arms of old people. Henoch–Schönlein purpura is a form of hypersensitivity angiitis giving skin purpura together with haematuria (due to a glomerulonephritis) and often abdominal pain due to intestinal purpura. It usually occurs in children and is frequently associated with a preceding streptococcal infection.

Platelet abnormalities may be quantitative or qualitative. Thrombocytopenic purpura is relatively common and results from many causes including leukaemia, lymphoma, severe infection, hypersensitivity reactions, hypersplenism, irradiation and cytotoxic drugs. The mechanism of the disorder may be decreased production, accelerated destruction or sequestration somewhere in the circulation. Defects in platelet function but with normal numbers are rare.

Haemophilia is the best known congenital disorder of the coagulation system. It is an X-linked recessive in which males suffer from the disease but females are asymptomatic carriers. The factor VIII deficiency results in bleeding, often into joints and soft tissue. It may complicate surgery or trauma by a continuous slow ooze from the wound. Christmas disease (factor IX deficiency) is clinically similar. Von Willebrand's disease is due to a defect in a platelet adhesion factor closely linked to factor VIII. It is inherited as an autosomal dominant and may give similar coagulation problems after surgery but joint involvement is rare.

Acquired coagulation disorders are seen especially in liver disease, for almost all the coagulation factors are made in hepatocytes. Circulating anticoagulants produce similar effects on the coagulation process. Obstructive jaundice leads to malabsorption of vitamin K (which is fat soluble and therefore needs bile salts for its absorption); this produces defects in prothrombin and factors VII, IX and X, giving a coagulation defect.

24

The Skeletal System

The joints

Acute arthritis

This may be bacterial in origin, developing through an open wound or by way of the bloodstream. In some cases suppuration may take place. The organisms most likely to cause the disease are the pyogenic cocci, particularly *staphylococcus aureus*. Gonococcal arthritis is now rare. Acute inflammation may also occur as a feature of some of the collagen diseases, such as rheumatic fever and anaphylactoid purpura, but in these instances mononuclear cells, rather than polymorphs, predominate. Another important cause of acute arthritis is associated with the precipitation of crystals into the synovium. Two conditions which commonly involve this process are *gout* (sodium urate crystals) and *pseudogout* (calcium pyrophosphate). Gout may occur as an hereditary disorder of purine metabolism or it may be secondary to rapid destruction of cell nuclei, as in the treatment of leukaemia. The acute arthritis most often affects the lower limb, particularly the metatarsal –phalangeal joint of the great toe.

Chronic bacterial arthritis

This may develop as a sequel of acute arthritis, or may be due to tuberculosis or syphilis. It is now a much rarer disease than it was at the beginning of the century, and this improvement is in large measure due to the success of antibiotic therapy.

Osteoarthritis

This is a common disease starting usually in late adult life, is insidious in onset, and chronic in progress. Men are more often affected than women, and the larger joints, especially the hip joint, are most frequently involved, giving rise to pain and limitation of movement. The aetiology is obscure; trauma may be an important initiating factor but the disease is commonly considered to be a degenerative process, first of cartilage and then bone. The joint cartilage loses its basophilia because mucopolysaccharides leak out. This reveals fibrillation of the matrix, the

225

fibrils running at right-angles to the articular surface. The surface cartilage splits along the fibrils and becomes roughened. Gradually it is worn away, exposing the underlying compact bone, which becomes smooth and hard due to new bone formation, and in places the surface is grooved. Beneath the sclerotic bone, trabeculae become osteoporotic and there is an excess of soft fibrous marrow with cysts in between, so that the bone may collapse at one or two points. New bone formation also takes place at the margin of the articular cartilage, leading to projections (osteophytes) which are usually capped by fibrocartilage. Villous projections may develop from the synovial membrane, consisting mainly of somewhat vascular fatty tissue, in which inflammatory cells are insignificant. Ankylosis or fusion of the joint surfaces does not take place. An extreme form of this degenerative joint disease is *Charcot's joint* which is associated with a neurological defect particularly seen in syphilis. This results in loss of sensation in the damaged joint.

Small bony projections on the terminal phalanges of the digits are common in old people (Heberden's nodes). They are disfiguring and may interfere with joint movement. Many regard them as mild foci of osteoarthritis, but this is by no means certain.

Rheumatoid arthritis

The essential features of the joint changes have been described previously (see p. 33). A similar arthritis is found in some patients with psoriasis and Reiter's syndrome (see p. 186).

Ankylosing spondylitis

The ligaments of the vertebrae in this disease undergo progressive ossification so that the movements of the spine become much reduced and eventually absent. The changes may involve the posterior intervertebral, costovertebral, and sacroiliac joints. The patients have a characteristic bowed and rigid posture. The disease appears to be allied to rheumatoid arthritis. Ninety per cent of patients with ankylosing spondylitis are HLA-B27 positive, compared with 8% of the general population. This clearly indicates a genetic predisposition to develop the disease.

Spinal osteophytosis

This disease is often misdiagnosed as spinal osteoarthritis. The osteophytes develop around vertebral bodies due to expansion of intervertebral discs as a result of degenerative disc disease. Osteoarthritis, being a disease of synovial joints, never affects the vertebral bodies. It may, however, affect the posterior intervertebral joints.

Tumours

Benign synoviomas (also known as giant cell tumours of tendon sheath and fibrous histiocytomas) occur particularly in tendon sheaths of the fingers and present as firm, brown nodules. About 20% of these tumours recur after excision. A similar histological appearance is found in pigmented villonodular synovitis which is believed to be a reactive proliferation of synovial tissue affecting principally the knee joint. Malignant synoviomas (synoviosarcomas) are rare tumours which occur usually around rather than in the larger joints of the lower limbs. They also occur between muscle planes, possibly arising from synovial bursae. They are destructive tumours and metastasize readily to the lungs.

The bones

Bones have three main functions: (a) the formation of a rigid framework for the body, (b) participation in the calcium and phosphorus metabolism of the body, and (c) the housing of the haemopoietic tissue. The disturbance of some of these functions has been considered in earlier chapters. The remainder will be mentioned here.

Metabolic bone disease

Bone consists of a fibrous matrix (osteoid) impregnated with calcium, magnesium, phosphate and carbonate to form hydroxyapatite. It is a labile tissue even in adults, calcium and phosphorus being laid down or absorbed according to need. Osteoblasts are flat or cuboidal cells lying close to the bone surface and are concerned mainly with bone formation. Osteoclasts are multinucleated giant cells derived from the bone marrow and scattered close to the bone surface. They are phagocytic cells and are active in absorption of bone. There are often notches in the bone adjacent to where they lie. Serum alkaline phosphatase activity is increased usually when there is increase of osteoblastic activity but the correlation is not exact. When studying bones histologically for evidence of metabolic activity, it has to be remembered that the usual preparations have been decalcified in order that they may be soft enough to cut. If it is required to determine how much calcium phosphate complex is present in the osteoid, undecalcified sections have to be prepared, a difficult technical procedure. Metabolic bone disease falls into two main groups: (1) disturbances in the osteoblast–osteoclast balance, and (2) disturbances in the mineralization of osteoid. The important examples of the first group are osteoporosis, osteosclerosis, osteitis fibrosa cystica (hyperparathyroidism) and osteitis deformans (Paget's disease). The second group consists in the main of the various manifestations of osteomalacia and rickets.

Osteoporosis

This consists of a reduction in the amount of bone without change in its chemical composition, i.e. the bone is of normal texture but there is less of it. Osteoporosis may be generalized or localized. The generalized form is most common in postmenopausal women. The total bone mass is maximal in both men and women during the third decade, and thereafter it declines. Oestrogen limits the loss of bone but after the menopause, when oestrogen levels fall, women suffer proportionately greater loss of bone. This may result in such weakening of the bone that fractures occur with minimal trauma. This is seen most often in vertebral bodies and in the femoral neck. Other causes of generalized osteoporosis include hyperthyroidism and Cushing's syndrome, both due to increased catabolic removal of bone. It may also be due to deficiency of protein or vitamin C (scurvy), the latter vitamin being necessary for the synthesis of the collagen matrix of bone. Examples of causes of localized osteoporosis are immobilization of the affected limb following nerve damage or fractures, and rheumatoid arthritis. For long it has been assumed that reduced bone formation is the important factor in the development of osteoporosis, but recent evidence has indicated that a long drawn-out, slightly increased bone resorption may be as important. A precise pathological diagnosis of the disease is difficult, because it is dependent on proving that the total mass of bone examined, though of normal texture, is of less volume than the normal counterpart. Radiological evidence of reduced cortical thickness of bone and multiple fractures, especially of vertebrae, are usually taken as the diagnostic features. The blood chemistry is normal.

Osteosclerosis

This is an increase in the mount of bone of normal chemical composition. It may occur if there is an excessive intake of fluoride (fluorosis) in the diet. However, the amount of fluorine added to municipal water supplies for protection against dental caries is always well below this toxic level. Abnormal bone may be produced, and result in osteosclerosis, in response to secondary carcinoma such as from prostate and breast, and hypertrophic osteoarthopathy which is a complication of cardiac and respiratory disorders. Because of the increased osteoblastic activity, the serum alkaline phosphatase may be increased.

Hyperparathyroidism

This may result from primary disease of the parathyroid glands such as adenoma, primary hyperplasia or carcinoma (see p. 209) or secondary hyperplasia associated with a low serum calcium level. The last-mentioned is most commonly due to an abnormality of vitamin D metabolism such as failure to synthesize the active form of the vitamin in the kidney, or lack of synthesis in the skin because of lack of exposure to sunlight. Malabsorption syndromes may also result in a failure to absorb sufficient calcium from the gut. Although the bone disease in both forms is similar, secondary hyperparathyroidism, in clinical practice, usually produces more severe disease as primary hyperparathyroidism is diagnosed and treated in most cases before severe bone disease has developed.

Hyperparathyroidism causes increased bone turnover. There is greatly increased osteoclastic resorption of bone and, at the same time, greatly increased osteoblastic bone formation. Usually the resorption predominates so that small subperiosteal erosions appear radiologically in bones such as those in the hand. The new bone which is formed is often 'woven' in pattern rather than being the normal 'lamellar' mature bone. Adjacent to the bone trabeculae, fibroblasts lay down collagen resulting in medullary fibrosis. In the most extreme forms of the disease, focal areas of total bone destruction may occur, the destroyed bone being replaced by fibrous tissue containing many osteoclasts. Radiologically, this appears as an area of increased lucency, misinterpreted as a bone cyst, and giving rise to the term *osteitis fibrosa cystica*.

Paget's disease of bone (osteitis deformans)

It has been known for some years that cases of Paget's disease occur more frequently in some areas, for example the North Midlands of England. More recently, inclusions resembling measles virus particles have been seen in osteoclasts associated with Paget's disease lesions. This raises the possibility of a viral aetiology for this disease. It is a disease mainly of the elderly; it may be widespread through the skeleton or localized to one bone. The bone is thickened, spongy and vascular. It is softer than normal and bends upon weight-bearing. Thickening of the bones results in compression of nerves passing through foramina in the skull and vertebral column causing pain and loss of function. The increased vascularity of the bones may have an effect similar to an arteriovenous aneurysm, causing a high cardiac output with subsequent cardiac failure. Histologically, the bones show increased osteoclastic resorption of normal dense cortical bone and osteoblastic deposition of abnormal trabeculae of new bone. This is deposited in an irregular fashion as shown by the mosaic pattern of cement lines. The medullary cavity is replaced by vascular fibrous tissue. Osteosarcoma develops in up to 10% of cases and represents 30% of all malignant primary tumours of bone in those over the age of 50.

Osteomalacia and rickets

The same pathological process operates in these two diseases, the differences that arise being attributable to the fact that rickets develops in the actively growing bones of childhood, whereas osteomalacia is the adult counterpart. The essential defect is that the osteoid stroma of the bone becomes imperfectly impregnated with calcium and phosphate, because there is an insufficient supply of these salts to the bones. The commonest cause of this is lack of vitamin D. Most vitamin D is synthesized in the skin from 7-dehydrocholesterol by the action of sunlight. It is transported to the liver, where 25-hydroxylation occurs, and from there to the kidney, where 1-hydroxylation produces the active form of the vitamin—1,25 dihydroxyvitamin D. A small quantity of vitamin D may be found in the diet, particularly in oily fish and in margarine to which it has been added. It undergoes similar hydroxylation in the liver and kidney. The vitamin is concerned with the maintenance of plasma calcium and phosphate levels by stimulating their intestinal absorption. It also stimulates renal tubular reabsorption of calcium and, with parathormone, mobilization of calcium and phosphate from bone. Where serum calcium and parathormone levels are normal, the renal 1-hydroxylation is switched to 24-hydroxylation to produce the apparently inactive 24,25-dihydroxyvitamin D.

Factors leading to osteomalacia include lack of exposure to sunlight, renal failure impairing the second hydroxylation of vitamin D, malabsorption of calcium and phosphate from the gut (e.g. postgastrectomy, coeliac disease, high fibre diet in Asians, and obstructive jaundice), some drugs which affect the metabolism of vitamin D, and hypophosphataemia which lowers the $Ca \times PO_4$ ion threshold in the blood and limits bone mineralization.

Failure of mineralization results in the bones being softer than normal. This is seen particularly in weight-bearing bones where deformity may be great. In children, the epiphyseal lines become widened and irregular as the cartilage cells survive for longer than normal. There is failure of provisional calcification in this cartilage. Capillaries grow into the cartilage from the metaphyseal end of the bone and bring with them osteoblasts which form osteoid. This also fails to calcify. Rickets is therefore best diagnosed by observing the wide, poorly ossifying, epiphyseal lines seen on x-ray; it can also be studied by costochrondral biopsy. The histological diagnosis of osteomalacia is dependent on demonstrating 'osteoid seams' at the edge of bone trabeculae in undecalcified sections. Not only are these seams wider and more extensive than normal, but the mineralization front is diminished or missing. This mineralization front lies at the interface of osteoid and mineralized bone and can be demonstrated by administering tetracycline to the patient before biopsy. The tetracycline is localized to the mineralization fronts and can be visualized by fluorescence microscopy.

Inflammation of bones

Osteomyelitis

This disease is much less common than before the days of antibiotic therapy, when it used to cause a high mortality and morbidity. The disease usually consists of a blood-borne infection such as *Staphylococcus aureus*, starting towards the end of the shaft of a long bone (metaphysis) and usually in young people. Compound fractures may also result in infection of bones. Suppuration results and, without active surgical drainage, is liable to spread both down the shaft of the bone and outwards, separating the periosteum from the underlying cortex. As a result, much of the bone becomes necrotic forming a 'sequestrum' which acts as a foreign body unless it is removed surgically or discharged spontaneously. The spontaneous discharge is often rendered difficult because the stripped periosteum starts to lay down new bone, often called an 'involucrum', which encases the sequestrum, albeit incompletely. Septicaemia may cause death within a few days. The long drawn-out suppuration following sequestrum formation used to be a frequent cause of amyloid disease. Extension into joints is uncommon.

Tuberculosis of bones and joints

This is again a disappearing disease because of improved social conditions and specific antibiotic therapy. It was in previous years an important cause of ill-health among the young. It is predominantly blood-borne and, in the old days, an appreciable fraction of cases was due to bovine tubercle bacilli ingested in infected milk. The joints may be involved primarily, or secondarily from bone, the avascular cartilage being no bar to the spread of tuberculosis, in contrast to the situation in acute osteomyelitis. Tubercles develop which lead to resorption and necrosis of bone and cartilage and disorganization of the joint cavity. Collapse and fracture of infected bone may occur, and the accumulating caseous material may spread into the surrounding tissues. The kyphosis and scoliosis of the spine resulting from tuberculous infection is often termed 'Pott's disease', and this may cause compression of the spinal cord and paraplegia. The local spread of infection from the vertebrae may track along the psoas muscle and present as a 'cold abscess' below the inguinal ligament.

Syphilis of bones and joints

This is again mainly of historical interest. Osteochondritis can form part of congenital syphilis. Chronic periostitis and gummatous necrosis are the commoner manifestations of tertiary syphilis, the former resulting in new bone formation giving, among other changes, 'sabre tibia' and the latter leading to the formation of cavities within the bone, the cranium and hard palate being relatively frequently involved.

Histiocytosis X

Eosinophilic granuloma is of unknown aetiology but it has the appearances of an inflammatory reaction. It causes destruction and expansion of bone, particularly in children. Local excision is usually curative. There are features of similarity with Hand–Schüller–Christian disease and Letterer–Siwe disease, so that the three are often grouped together under the term Histiocytosis X.

Fractures

The processes involved in the repair of fractured bones have already been briefly outlined (see p. 19).

Tumours

Secondary tumours, usually carcinomas, are much commoner than primary malignant tumours of bone. Certain carcinomas show a predilection for metastasizing to bone and these include carcinoma of the lung, breast, prostate, thyroid and kidney.

Primary tumours of bone: benign

Osteoid osteoma is a tumour of adolescents and young adults. It occurs in the shaft of long bones and presents as bone pain. Radiologically, the lesion is osteolytic surrounded by a rim of sclerotic bone. It consists of immature, woven bone and osteoid matrix. A similar, but larger lesion may be found in vertebrae and is called *benign osteoblastoma*.

Exostosis develops from *ecchondroma* by ossification. These are developmental abnormalities rather than true tumours. They arise on the outer aspect of long bones near the epiphyseal cartilage and may produce large masses that limit movement of adjacent joints. They rarely become malignant but when they do so it tends to be those that occur in the proximal parts of the limb. Multiple ecchondromas and exostoses are called *diaphyseal aclasis*, which is inherited as a dominant gene.

Enchondroma is a cartilage tumour occurring most commonly in the shaft of long bones, the metacarpals, metatarsals and phalanges often being involved. Tumours occurring in the distal part of the limb almost never become malignant but tumours in the humerus, femur or limb girdles may do so, forming chondrosarcoma.

Fibrous dysplasia of bone may present as a tumour but is another developmental abnormality. It consists of fibrous tissue arranged in a whorled pattern and contains spicules of woven bone. The lesion may be single or multiple, the latter sometimes associated with skin pigmentation and precocious puberty (especially in females), giving *Albright's syndrome*.

Other benign tumours in bone include angiomas and neurofibromas similar to their counterparts in soft tissues.

Giant cell tumour of bone (osteoclastoma) falls between benign and malignant tumours. After local excision, about half of these tumours behave as benign neoplasms but, of the remainder, two-thirds will be locally invasive and one-third metastasize to lungs. Osteoclastomas rarely occur under the age of 20. They are found in the ends of long bones as osteolytic lesions which may show pathological fracture. The tumour has two components, a multinucleate giant cell resembling osteoclasts and a background spindle cell. It is this background cell which is the better guide to malignancy as assessed by mitotic activity and pleomorphism.

Primary tumours of bone: malignant

Although primary malignant tumours of bone account for only 1% of deaths from malignancy, they are relatively common amongst sarcomas, especially in children. By far the most important and the commonest is *osteosarcoma*. This occurs most frequently in the second decade of life, although Paget's disease of bone gives rise to some cases in later life. The tumours occur most frequently around the growing ends of long bones, particularly those around the knee. They may be osteolytic or osteosclerotic. The periosteum is raised by the expanding tumour, and this periosteum lays down new bone. Histologically, there may be a mixture of cartilage, fibrous tissue and bone, but in all osteosarcomas there is evidence of osteoid formation by malignant cells. Osteosarcomas metastasize readily by the bloodstream to the lungs and there is a very poor five-year survival. A variant, known as *parosteal osteosarcoma*, grows from the external surface of the bone and is usually very well differentiated. It is separated from the others because of its better prognosis.

Chondrosarcoma occurs later in life than osteosarcoma and affects the proximal ends of long bones, the limb girdles and ribs. The tumour consists entirely of cartilage and this shows all degrees of differentiation. These tumours are more slow growing than osteosarcoma and usually can be treated locally, although eventually they metastasize to lungs.

Giant cell tumour of bone has been described on p. 232.

Ewing's tumour is a tumour of childhood and young adult life; it arises from the medullary cavity of the bone. It is non-osteogenic and consists of small, dark-staining cells which destroy the bone. When the bone expands there may be some reactive (not tumorous) periosteal new bone formation. The tumour is rapidly growing and metastasizes by the bloodstream to lungs, liver and to other parts of the skeleton. It may be difficult to distinguish these tumours from metastatic neuroblastoma.

Malignant lymphoma may arise as a primary tumour of the medullary cavity in adults. There is destruction of bone but these tumours are not as aggressive as osteosarcomas and they may show a good response to radiotherapy. Malignant lymphoma and leukaemia may also affect the bones as part of a widespread disease affecting many organs of the body. Myeloma has already been discussed (see p. 222).

Malignant tumours of bone also include fibrosarcoma arising from periosteum or nerve sheath, liposarcoma and angiosarcoma.

Chordoma is a locally malignant tumour that arises from the remains of the notochord. It occurs more in older individuals at the lower or upper end of the vertebral column and consists of gelatinous masses of tissue with areas of haemorrhage and necrosis. Metastases are rare.

Adamantinoma (ameloblastoma) is a tumour found mainly in the lower jaw and is formed from the enamel organ of teeth. It consists of islands of epithelial cells in a fibrous stroma, the outer layers of the islands being columnar or cuboidal, resembling basal cell carcinoma, and the inner layers being loose textured pale cells—the stellate reticulum. These tumours are locally infiltrative and destructive, causing expansion of bone, but they rarely metastasize.

Voluntary muscles

Atrophy

Atrophy of muscles takes place if they are immobilized, if there has been prolonged bedrest, or if there is paralysis of the nerve of supply. It may also follow inanition or cachexia, and is a prominent feature of primary muscle diseases (myopathies).

Hypertrophy

This can follow exercise; it may be compensatory, following atrophy of adjacent muscle fibres in neuromuscular diseases.

Myositis ossificans

This state is liable to develop if there has been haematoma formation in traumatized muscle near to bone, and consists of ectopic ossification in the organizing lesion.

Muscular dystrophies

This is a group of genetic disorders affecting different groups of muscles and leading to progressive weakness. Histologically, a number of degenerative changes occur in individual muscle fibres. The three principal varieties of muscular dystrophy are *pseudohypertrophic muscular dystrophy* (Duchenne), *facio-scapulo-humeral muscular dystrophy* and *dystrophia myotonica*. The first is inherited as a sex-linked recessive, affecting males in the first years of life. The diseased muscles are mainly in the lower limbs. The term pseudohypertrophic refers to the enlargement of the muscle due to adipose tissue replacement. The facio-scapulo-humeral variety is inherited as an autosomal dominant and occurs in older children and young adults. Its name describes its distribution; the onset of the disease is usually insidious and it affects both males and females. Dystrophia myotonica affects both sexes and has a dominant inheritance. Clinical disease typically develops in adult life and is associated with cataracts, testicular atrophy and baldness. The myotonia produces both slow contraction and slow relaxation of the affected muscle.

The distinction between these dystrophies and myositis may be difficult. Muscular dystrophies can usually be distinguished from neural atrophy in which damaged nerves and whole bundles of atrophic muscle fibres can be seen. An increase of fat may be present among the atrophied muscle fibres.

Myasthenia gravis

Myasthenia gravis leads to marked muscular weakness as a result of an abnormal response of the motor end-plates in the muscle. It is now recognized that the abnormality is an autoimmune disease with antibodies directed against acetylcholine receptors, inhibiting neuromuscular transmission. The muscle weakness can be abolished by administering anticholinesterase drugs such as neostigmine. Collections of lymphocytes (lymphorrhages) are found in the muscle. In 10–15% of cases, particularly in patients over the age of 30, there is an associated thymoma, and in almost all other cases there is thymic hyperplasia. Thymectomy is undertaken as a therapeutic procedure in this disease.

Myositis

Inflammation of muscle may be associated with a neighbouring pyogenic infection or it may be due to tuberculosis, sarcoid, virus infections, parasites, or 'collagen diseases' such as dermatomyositis, scleroderma, polyarteritis nodosa or rheumatoid arthritis.

Tumours

These are rare. *Rhabdomyoma* may be found in cardiac muscle but primary neoplasms of voluntary muscle are all malignant. Rhabdomyosarcomas are of several types; most occur in childhood and early adult life. A form which occurs in young children is the embryonal rhabdomyosarcoma. These tend to occur in such sites as bladder, prostate, vagina, palate and orbit. They may grow as grape-like tumours (botryoid). In adults, rhabdomyosarcomas develop more often in large muscle masses. They produce tumours with gross nuclear pleomorphism and bizarre tumour giant cells. All forms of rhabdomyosarcoma are highly malignant.

25

The Central Nervous System

General pathology

A neuron consists of nucleus and cytoplasm like other cells. The cytoplasm of the cell body contains basophilic granules of RNA (Nissl granules). Cell processes (dendrites) arise from the cell body and there is a prolonged process (the axon) which, with other axons, makes up nerves. If the continuity of a nerve is interrupted, the distal part undergoes degeneration, i.e. it swells and then becomes absorbed. Myelin sheaths break up into a number of fatty globules. The cell body also undergoes degenerative changes referred to as axonal reaction. The Nissl granules in the perinuclear cytoplasm disappear (chromatolysis), there is swelling of the cell cytoplasm and displacement of the nucleus to the periphery of the cell. If the cell dies, the nucleus undergoes karyolysis. Damaged nerve cells are capable of recovery but new ones cannot be formed. If the fibrous sheath of the distal part of the axon remains close to the proximal end, regeneration of the nerve can take place by growth of the axon from the proximal end into the distal sheath. At times, overgrowth of divided nerves and their fibrous sheaths gives rise to small, painful nodules called traumatic neuromas. Regeneration rarely happens in the brain and spinal cord where there is no neurilemmal sheath for the axon. The power of regeneration is therefore practically confined to peripheral axons.

Neuroglia forms the supporting framework of the neurons in the brain and spinal cord. It is made up of three types of cells: astrocytes, oligodendrocytes and microglia. Ependyma may also be included. Astrocytes are of two types, protoplasmic astrocytes with short branching processes found in the grey matter and fibrous astrocytes with longer processes and fewer branches found in the white matter. The long processes of fibrous astrocytes contain glial fibres. Protoplasmic astrocytes can convert to the fibrous type around sites of injury and produce these intracellular fibres (gliosis). Gliosis is the main repair process in the central nervous system, corresponding to fibrosis elsewhere. It consists largely of the proliferation of these fibrous astrocytes. There is little fibrous connective tissue in the brain but true fibrosis does occur where tissue destruction is extensive. Fibroblasts from perivascular connective tissue proliferate and produce collagen which is then found in the damaged area. Oligodendrocytes occur around neurons and along their axons. They appear to have a nutritive function. Around damaged neurons they may swell and become more numerous—satellitosis. Microglia differs from the other glial cells in that it is not of neuroectodermal origin but is a mesodermal histiocyte. It is phagocytic and may take up lipid, becoming foamy, when it is referred to as a *compound granular corpuscle*.

Necrosis of central nervous tissue, if at all extensive and sudden, is followed by liquefaction, so that softening and ultimately cyst formation occur. Inflammatory cells of repair are derived from the bloodstream. The dead tissue is phagocytosed by histiocytes from the blood and by microglia. Surrounding this there is a scar consisting of glial fibres and collagen.

Central nervous tissue can become oedematous but the oedema is mainly intracellular. There is astrocytic swelling, splitting of the myelin lamellae and dilatation of perivascular spaces. The white matter appears swollen and moist, there is widening of the gyri and flattening of the brain surface where it is compressed against the skull. Histologically, the tissue appears more reticulated than normal. Rise of intracranial pressure will give papilloedema and retinal haemorrhages. There will be herniation of the cerebellar tonsils into the foramen magnum, compressing the medullary centres of respiration and circulation, herniation of the uncinate gyrus through the incisura of the tentorium cerebelli and, if there is unilateral swelling of a cerebral hemisphere, herniation of the cingulate gyrus under the falx cerebri. Herniation of the brain is more likely to occur if there is a sudden rise of intracranial pressure or if cerebrospinal fluid is withdrawn by lumbar puncture.

Congenital malformations

Anencephaly is a failure of development of the brain and is often accompanied by failure of closure of the neural tube—rachischisis—which may be partial or complete. The mildest degree of failure of closure affects only the vertebral arches, usually in the lumbar region, and gives rise to spina bifida occulta. The underlying cord is usually in the correct position. A meningocele occurs when failure of spinal fusion is accompanied by protrusion of the meninges, meningomyelocele when there is protrusion of the cord and meninges, and syringomyelocele when there is dilatation of the spinal canal in association with the defect in the vertebral arches. Encephalocele occurs when there is a defect in the midline of the occiput. The Arnold–Chiari malformation consists of herniation of the venteromedial portion of the cerebellum, the fourth ventricle and the medulla into the foramen magnum resulting in hydrocephalus. This malformation is often accompanied by other congenital defects such as stenosis of the aqueduct, platybasia (flattening of the base of the skull resulting in narrowing of the foramen magnum),

Klippel–Feil abnormality (fusion of the cervical vertebrae), fusion of the atlas to the occiput, and spina bifida. The Arnold–Chiari malformation may not become apparent until adult life.

Hydrocephalus

Cerebrospinal fluid is secreted into the lateral ventricles by the choroid plexus and circulates through the third ventricle into the fourth ventricle, from which it escapes by way of the foramina of Luschka and Magendie into the subarachnoid space. The fluid is mainly absorbed through arachnoid granulations into the venous sinuses. Obstruction to the normal flow of cerebrospinal fluid leads to dilatation of the ventricular system—hydrocephalus. It is called communicating if there is access from the ventricles to the spinal subarachnoid space but not to the cerebral subarachnoid space, i.e. the obstruction must be at the base of the brain, and non-communicating if the whole subarachnoid space is blocked from the ventricles, i.e. the obstruction must be within the ventricular system. The commonest sites of obstruction to cerebrospinal fluid circulation are the aqueduct of Sylvius and the subarachnoid space around the base of the brain. Hydrocephalus can be congenital or acquired. In the congenital form, obstruction can occur at many sites, though 50% of cases arise as a result of stenosis of the aqueduct. Other causes include the Arnold–Chiari malformation and intrauterine infections such as toxoplasmosis. Tumours pressing on the aqueduct rarely give congenital hydrocephalus. The ventricles may become enormously dilated and the fontanelles of the skull widely separated. Functional disturbance may be much less than would be expected from the degree and duration of the ventricular dilatation. Acquired hydrocephalus may result from (a) pressure on the aqueduct by tumour, or (b) meningitic occlusion of the arachnoid cisterns at the base of the brain. As the suture lines are often closed in this type of hydrocephalus, the brain becomes compressed against the skull and there is rapid destruction of brain tissue.

Syringomyelia

This disease is of uncertain aetiology. The cord is most commonly enlarged in the cervical region by a cyst containing yellow fluid and surrounded by glial scar tissue. The cyst does not communicate with the spinal canal and is not lined by ependyma. Pressure on the sensory and later the motor pathways leads to loss of sensation, especially for heat and pain, and upper motor neuron signs in the legs. Charcot's joint may develop in the shoulder.

The effects of trauma

A number of lesions may develop from trauma. Concussion may occur following blunt trauma without evidence of gross lesions, but there is experimental evidence that there is damage to cells in the brainstem and cerebral cortex. With more severe injuries, damage to the brain in the form of punctate haemorrhages and oedema (contusion) may be observed in two sites: (1) immediately beneath the point of impact, and (2) at the diametrically opposite pole (*contre-coup*). The latter is more frequent and more severe than the former. Laceration of the brain with rupture of membranes may also occur and there may be fractures of the adjacent bone. An important form of haemorrhage is an *extradural haemorrhage* usually associated with skull fracture and rupture of a branch of the middle meningeal artery. There may be transient loss of consciousness followed by a lucid interval, and then a second deepening phase of unconsciousness associated with a rise of intracranial pressure which can be relieved by timely surgical intervention. *Subdural haemorrhage* may be acute or chronic. Acute haemorrhages are usually due to tearing of the arachnoid, often associated with laceration of the brain. Chronic subdural haemorrhage results from the rupture of bridging veins in the subdural space resulting in the slow leakage of blood. This undergoes organization to form a mass which compresses the brain. Chronic subdural haematomas used to be thought of as a manifestation of syphilis due to their frequency in patients with general paralysis of the insane (GPI), but these haematomas are now recognized as being traumatic. *Subarachnoid haemorrhage* may also result from trauma.

Infection may be introduced into the cerebrospinal fluid or brain by penetrating wounds.

Intracerebral haemorrhage

Massive cerebral haemorrhage, which is a cause of 'stroke', is a common, usually progressive, and therefore fatal illness among older patients. Hypertension and atherosclerosis are the common associated conditions. The haemorrhage is found most frequently in the lentiform nucleus due to rupture of the lenticulostriate branch of the middle cerebral artery. Pontine haemorrhages may occur spontaneously or they may be secondary to cerebral haemorrhage with displacement of the brain downwards. It can be shown by microangiography that small aneurysms develop in intracerebral arteries in hypertensive patients, and rupture of these arteries is believed to be the basis of cerebral haemorrhage in hypertension. Other causes of cerebral haemorrhage include trauma, angiomatous malformation, tumour, haemorrhagic diathesis, fat embolism, asphyxia, severe infections and vitamin B deficiency. The haemorrhages in many of these conditions are multiple and petechial.

Subarachnoid haemorrhage

Apart from trauma, causes of subarachnoid haemorrhage are rupture of a congenital 'berry' aneurysm (see p. 116), and extension of an intracerebral haemorrhage into the subarachnoid space. Rarely, mycotic or atheromatous aneurysms of the circle of Willis may rupture. Blood mixes with the cerebrospinal fluid, initially causing meningeal irritation but later causing a rise in intracranial pressure leading to coma and death. Blood-stained cerebrospinal fluid from a subarachnoid haemorrhage may be distinguished from a bloody tap due to perforation of a vertebral vein during lumbar puncture by the uniform distribution of blood and the yellow (xanthochromic) staining of the supernatant fluid after centrifugation of the former.

Cerebral infarction

This is another common cause of 'stroke'. It is usually due to atheroma and follows occlusion of a branch of one of the cerebral arteries, often the middle cerebral artery. It may also be due to occlusion of the internal carotid artery by atheroma or thrombus. Embolism from an atheromatous plaque, or from the heart due to atrial fibrillation or mural thrombus following myocardial infarction, will have a similar result. Less commonly, cerebral infarction may be due to polyarteritis nodosa. A cerebral infarct softens quickly and eventually becomes cystic. There is gliosis around the infarcted area and slight brown staining due to haemosiderin deposition. Microscopically, degenerate tissue is seen to be phagocytosed by microglia which accumulate cytoplasmic lipid to form cells called compound granular corpuscles. Cerebral infarction may cause death before these changes have had sufficient time to develop.

Thrombosis of spinal arteries may follow compression due to fractured vertebrae, tumour or abscess, or it may be due to syphilitic endarteritis. Infarction of the spinal cord causes paraplegia due to interruption of the long tracts.

Infection of brain and spinal cord

Infections of the brain, spinal cord and meninges may be due to bacteria, viruses, spirochaetes, fungi, protozoa and worms. The complications of bacterial infection are much less common than in former days because of a favourable response to early antibiotic treatment.

Suppurative meningitis

The commonest organisms are pneumococci, meningococci and

Haemophilus influenzae. Infection reaches the meninges through the bloodstream, most commonly from the lungs, although infection may also spread direct from the middle ear or penetrating wounds. In pneumococcal infection, the inflammatory reaction and exudate are most noticeable over the convex surface of the cerebral hemispheres, but in other infections the base of the brain is more severely affected. Microscopically, polymorphs and fibrinous exudate fill the subarachnoid space and extend around the vessels into the brain in the Virchow–Robin spaces. Many polymorphs will be found in a specimen of CSF.

Tuberculous meningitis

Tuberculous meningitis is usually a result of miliary tuberculosis. The exudate is serofibrinous and predominantly basal. Small miliary tubercles can be identified, especially along the middle cerebral artery. A small cortical 'tuberculoma'—Rich's focus—may also be identified. The cellular infiltrate is atypical for tuberculosis in that it rarely shows caseation or Langhans-type giant cells. There is a predominance of lymphocytes in the infiltrate and in the CSF. There is endarteritis obliterans. Healing may leave fibrous obliteration of the subarachnoid space and result in hydrocephalus (see p. 238).

Cerebral abscess

This may result from direct spread of infection from the middle ear or paranasal air sinuses, from penetrating wounds or from blood-borne infection, especially from bronchiectasis and bacterial endocarditis. Patients present most frequently with signs of raised intracranial pressure and localizing signs according to the site involved. Macroscopically, there is destruction of brain tissue with accumulation of pus and surrounding gliosis. There is progressive spread of the infection unless it is treated.

Virus infections

There are many virus infections of the central nervous system and they may produce their effects directly by damaging cells or indirectly via immunological mechanisms. Infection may involve predominantly the meninges (meningitis), the brain (encephalitis), or the spinal cord (myelitis). There may be overlap in the structures involved and such terms as meningoencephalitis and encephalomyelitis are used.

Aseptic meningitis is a syndrome characterized by fever, meningism and a raised lymphocyte count in the cerebrospinal fluid. Echo and Coxsackie viruses are responsible for many cases, but other viruses (such as the arena virus of lymphocytic choriomeningitis) can produce a similar picture. Tuberculosis, leptospirosis and cryptococcosis may also produce these changes.

In most instances a viraemia precedes the neurological symptoms; there is congestion of the meninges with lymphocytic infiltration. Recovery occurs in all but a few cases.

Viral encephalitis

Encephalitis is usually taken to mean a non-suppurative inflammation of the brain. Three patterns of disease are recognized.

1. *Primary*, where the brain is the major organ involved and is directly damaged by a virus, usually transmitted from an animal. Clinically there is a raised temperature, dysfunction of the brain, a raised cerebrospinal fluid pressure, and lymphocytosis. In the brain there is: (a) destruction of nerve cells bodies, (b) perivascular collections of lymphocytes and plasma cells, (c) proliferation of microglia, and (d) sometimes characteristic inclusion bodies such as the cytoplasmic Negri bodies of rabies.

Mosquito- and tick-borne arboviruses are major causes of encephalitis world wide. Rabies follows a bite from an infected animal. The virus appears to travel along nerves and then to multiply in the grey matter. The incubation period is usually one to two months but may be up to a year. The disease is almost invariably fatal once clinical manifestations have developed. Encephalitis lethargica is included in this group, though no virus has been identified.

2. *Secondary* encephalitis occurs as an occasional complication of some systemic diseases. Thus it can follow bacterial, spirochaetal, parasitic, rickettsial or other viruses such as herpes or Coxsackie. Pathological changes are usually similar to those of the primary group.

3. *Postinfectious* encephalitis is an occasional result of a systemic viral infection, particularly the common exanthemata such as measles and rubella. Clinically the disease is like other acute encephalitides. Pathologically, the prominent lesion is perivascular lymphocytic cuffing. These diseases are believed to be hypersensitivity reactions similar to those seen in animals in experimental allergic encephalomyelitis. Most of the patients recover but there is an appreciable mortality.

Myelitis

Poliomyelitis is the most important viral infection of the spinal cord, though prophylaxis has dramatically reduced its incidence in developed countries. It is an enterovirus. After an incubation period of 10 days there are systemic symptoms of malaise, sore throat and vomiting and neurological manifestations of headache, stiff neck and limb pains. These are followed by flaccid paralysis of affected muscles. The infection may abort at any stage. In the acute stage the cord is congested and microscopically there is perivascular inflammatory cell cuffing and degeneration of the motor neurons of the anterior horns. In long-term survivors there may be gliosis in the anterior horns.

Unusual virus infections

Typically, a neurotropic virus has a short incubation period, a rapid onset and course, leading either to death or, if antibodies develop and the virus is eliminated, to recovery. *Latent* (or *persistent*) virus infections are those in which the virus is present but is not manifest or active. Herpes zoster in an active phase produces a vesicular eruption of the skin in the distribution of the involved nerve. In the latent phase, the virus lives in the dorsal root ganglion of the nerve. Factors which precipitate activation are not well understood. Herpes simplex and the virus of subacute sclerosing panencephalitis also can be latent.

Slow viruses are those with very long incubation periods (many years). The first examples were described in animals, but in man, kuru (a disease formerly associated with cannibalism in the Highlands of New Guinea) was shown to be due to a transmissible agent being eaten. Jakob–Creutzfeldt disease (previously classified as a degenerative disorder) has also been shown to be due to a virus. In both kuru and Jakob–Creutzfeldt disease there is dementia associated with progressive neuronal loss and gliosis. The most characteristic change in Jakob–Creutzfeldt disease is spongiosis, a neurocystic degenerative change; it is best to refer to this disorder as spongiform encephalopathy.

Neurosyphilis

Formerly, up to 10% of patients with untreated syphilis used to die of central nervous system manifestations, but death from these complications is rare today.

Meningovascular syphilis usually develops in the first three years of the primary infection. There is chronic inflammation of the meninges over the convex surface of the cerebral hemispheres, the meninges appearing opaque. There is also an endarteritis obliterans of the vessels which may give small infarcts; in the spinal cord it may lead to transverse myelitis and paraplegia.

Tabes dorsalis and *general paresis* are late manifestations of syphilis. In tabes, the manifestations include ataxia, lightening pains, loss of sensation, optic atrophy and Argyll Robertson pupils. There may be an associated severe osteoarthritis (Charcot's joints). The most obvious neurological lesion is atrophy of the dorsal aspects of the cord, but the basic pathology is in the root entry zones where the dorsal roots entering the cord are covered with oligodendrocytes rather than Schwann cells. Here, there are meningovascular lesions which cause damage to the axons. Tabes is therefore a late form of meningovascular syphilis. In *general paresis* there is loss of intellect, personality changes, inco-ordination, hyperactive reflexes, eye changes and focal neurological lesions. There is cortical atrophy and thickening of the meninges; neurons, blood vessels and meninges are involved. This is truly parenchymatous syphilis. A *gumma* can occur in the central nervous system.

Though different types of neurosyphilis are described, it is one disease, with overlapping manifestations.

Fungal infections

Fungal infections of the brain and meninges are rare and usually fatal. They are seen particularly in patients on immunosuppressive therapy or with advanced malignant disease. One of the most important in Britain is infection with *Cryptococcus neoformans* which produces meningitis. The meninges may be thickened and opaque, resembling tuberculous meningitis. The encapsulated organisms are usually profuse but there is little cellular reaction to them. Other fungal infections include histoplasmosis, coccidiodomycosis and actinomycosis.

Protozoal infections

Toxoplasmosis is important as a cause of encephalitis *in utero* and in the newborn. There is inflammation of the meninges and brain substance, resulting in hydrocephalus and cerebral calcification. The disease in the mother escapes detection although antibodies may be demonstrated in the maternal serum.

Cerebral malaria due to *P. falciparum* (see p. 38) and trypanosomiasis (see p. 40) are also examples of cerebral protozoal infections.

Worm infestations

Cysticercosis (caused by the larval form of *Taenia solium*) and hydatid cysts (*Echinococcus granulosus*) may involve the brain. *Toxocara canis* produces granulomatous inflammation in the brain and in the retina. In trichinosis (*Trichinella spiralis*) the parasite may block small arterioles, causing an acute inflammatory reaction with many eosinophils.

Demyelinating diseases

Demyelination is seen as degeneration and disappearance of the myelin sheaths of the axons in the central nervous system. It occurs as a consequence of destruction of axons in many disorders, when it is called secondary demyelination. In the primary demyelinating disorders, the axons remain intact initially though they are damaged later. *Multiple sclerosis* is the most important of these diseases. It typically starts in young adults and usually runs a downhill course with exacerbations and remissions and neurological lesions separated in time and space. The lesions are seen as plaques of demyelination anywhere in the central nervous system but especially in the white matter around the posterior horns of the lateral ventricles. They are often centred on a venule where lymphocyte cuffing is seen. There is demyelination and infiltration with macrophages. Gliosis follows and axons disappear from advanced lesions. The cause of this disorder is unknown; there is an increased frequency of HLA-A3, -BR7 and -DR2 in patients but it is likely that an environmental agent is more important than heredity in its aetiology. There are some rarer disorders which are clinically different but have similar pathology to multiple sclerosis. These include *diffuse cerebral sclerosis* (Schilder's disease), *concentric sclerosis* (Balo's disease), and *optic neuromyelopathy* (Devic's disease). The *postinfectious encephalomyelopathies* are rare complications of several common viral diseases, e.g. measles and mumps. The lesions show demyelination, haemorrhage, lymphocytes and polymorphs. They are found around veins and venules, especially in the pons and the white matter of the cerebrum and cerebellum.

Deficiency disorders occur in the absence of vital nutrients. *Subacute combined degeneration of the cord* is a serious complication of pernicious anaemia. Vitamin B_{12} deficiency results in demyelination of the posterior and lateral columns of the cord without subsequent gliosis. The most common symptoms of the disease are paraesthesiae in the hands and feet with loss of vibration sense. Later there may be spasticity of the limbs as a result of upper motor neuron involvement.

Wernicke's encephalopathy is due to thiamine deficiency. It is seen particularly in alcoholics where it results in ocular abnormalities, mental changes and ataxia. The lesions are found in the mammillary bodies, the walls of the third ventricle, aqueduct and fourth ventricle. They consist of brown discoloration and haemorrhages associated with endothelial proliferation of small vessels.

Pellagra is associated with abnormalities of tryptophan metabolism and associated nicotinic acid deficiency. The classical triad of dermatitis, dementia and diarrhoea is seen. In the brain there is loss of ganglion cells in the cortex, basal ganglia and also the anterior horn cells of the cord. Pellegra is commonly part of a mixed deficiency in people with a poor diet.

Metabolic abnormalities

There are many inborn errors of metabolism affecting the nervous system. The *leucodystrophies* are abnormalities of myelin leading to deficient myelination and axonal degeneration in all parts of the central nervous system. Most of them have an autosomal recessive inheritance. The *storage diseases* such as Tay–Sachs and Niemann–Pick result from lysosomal enzyme deficiencies causing cells to accumulate material which they cannot metabolize. Most of the these disorders are also autosomal recessives.

Copper accumulates in the central nervous system and liver in *Wilson's disease* and causes hepatolenticular degeneration. Many *toxins* produce lesions in the CNS.

Degenerative diseases

There are many disorders of the central nervous system which are characterized by nerve cell loss, reactive gliosis and demyelination when myelinated axons are destroyed. Some of these occur in well-recognized clinical patterns with a characteristic distribution of lesions often involving one particular neural system. Examples of these disorders are given below, with the predominant system involved given first.

Cerebral

Diffuse cerebral atrophy may be the cause of senile dementia. Similar pathology is seen in *Alzheimer's disease*, which is its presenile equivalent. There may be deposits of amyloid in the brain in these diseases. In *Pick's disease*, another presenile dementia, the cerebral atrophy is focal.

Cerebellar

In *spinocerebellar* and *olivopontocerebellar degeneration* there is progressive development of ataxia. A similar process is seen in the cerebellar degeneration sometimes occurring with a carcinoma elsewhere in the body.

Extrapyramidal system

Parkinson's disease is characterized by tremor, rigidity and slowness of movement. Classically, it develops in elderly people and is of unknown aetiology (paralysis agitans). Some cases follow encephalitis, some are associated with arteriosclerosis, and there are some drug-induced cases (especially associated with phenothiazines). In addition to the usual features of a degenerative disorder, there is loss of pigmented cells from the substantia nigra; biochemical studies have shown that there is dopamine depletion in these areas.

Motor

Progressive muscle weakness develops in *motor neuron disease* and its variants. The precise features depend on whether the upper or lower motor neurons are predominantly involved and in what combination.

Visual

Loss of vision is the major feature of two hereditary disorders, *retinitis pigmentosum* and *hereditary optic atrophy*. There is usually little evidence of lesions elsewhere in the central nervous system.

Though some of these degenerative disorders have a strong hereditary basis, the aetiology and pathogenesis of most are obscure.

Tumours

Primary tumours of the brain are less common than secondary tumours, the most important metastatic tumours in the brain being from carcinoma of the lung and breast. Metastatic deposits of carcinoma are most commonly situated in the cerebral hemisphere at the junction of the grey and white matter. They are usually multiple, well defined, and reproduce the histological features of the primary tumour. Haemorrhage into the necrotic centre of the tumour is a common terminal event. Cerebellar metastases are about half as common as those in the cerebral hemispheres. Metastatic tumour in the meninges may result in seedling deposits throughout the subarachnoid space. The CSF will have a raised cell count and tumour cells may be identified.

Glioma

Astrocytoma accounts for most gliomas. It arises anywhere in the brain or spinal cord but is found most frequently in the cerebral hemispheres in adults and in the cerebellum in children. The tumour may become cystic and this is seen most often in the childhood cerebellar tumours. Haemorrhage and necrosis are common in the more malignant varieties. Astrocytomas may be graded according to their degree of differentiation, but this varies in different parts of the tumour and grading may be misleading in small diagnostic biopsies. The best differentiated are ill-defined tumours that may produce increased firmness of the brain and enlargement of one hemisphere. The edge of the tumour may be impossible to identify and histologically there may be great difficulty in distinguishing this from reactive gliosis. These tumours tend to recur after attempted excision and cause death usually within a few years. At the other end of the scale, highly malignant astrocytomas show greatly increased cellularity, pleomorphism, mitoses and vascular proliferation with prominent endothelial cells. These highly malignant tumours used to be called *glioblastoma multiforme*. They may reach massive size and cause death within a few months of diagnosis. Haemorrhage and necrosis are features of these more malignant tumours.

Oligodendroglioma is very much less common than astrocytoma. It occurs in adults, usually in the frontal lobes, and is rare in children. These tumours tend to be well differentiated and slow growing with focal areas of calcification which may facilitate their radiological localization. Less commonly, more malignant variants may be impossible to distinguish from other highly malignant gliomas. Histologically, these tumours consist of neat, box-like cells with clear cytoplasm giving a honeycomb appearance.

Ependymoma is a slow-growing tumour that occurs mostly in children and young adults. It arises from the walls of the ventricles or spinal canal, most commonly the fourth ventricle. Most of these tumours consist of epithelioid cells arranged in rosettes. A papillary pattern of growth may be found and this is often accompanied by a myxomatous stroma—myxopapillary ependymoma. These papillary tumours should be distinguished from benign choroidal papillomas which are common in children and may cause hydrocephalus. Papillomas are difficult to remove and as a result they may recur.

Medulloblastoma is a tumour confined to children. It arises in the midline of the cerebellum from primitive neural tissue before differentiation into neurons and glia. The tumour consists of small dark-staining cells resembling adrenal neuroblastomas and retinoblastomas. Because medulloblastomas are situated near the fourth ventricle there is a risk of obstruction to the flow of CSF resulting in hydrocephalus. These tumours have a very poor prognosis.

Spread of gliomas

Medulloblastomas show the greatest tendency to metastasize through the subarachnoid space. Other gliomas, even the more highly malignant varieties, do not metastasize outside the central nervous system unless there has been surgical intervention when they may involve the skull and tissues of the neck. They are all locally invasive within the brain and cord.

Vascular tumours

Vascular malformations (angiomas) in the brain and meninges may be a cause of cerebral haemorrhage. The only true vascular tumour of any importance is the *haemangioblastoma*. This is a cystic cerebellar tumour, found mostly in children. In the wall of the cyst there is usually a nodule consisting of endothelial-lined vascular spaces and lipid-laden foamy cells. These tumours are always well circumscribed and therefore more amenable to surgery than most cerebral tumours. Haemangioblastoma may be associated with retinal angioma and cystic disease of the pancreas and kidney (Lindau–von Hippel disease).

Meningioma

These tumours arise from arachnoid cells that protude into dural venous sinuses. The most common sites are along the superior saggital sinus, the sphenoidal ridge, the olfactory groove, the posterior cranial fossa, and along the spinal cord. They are slow-growing, well-defined tumours that compress surrounding structures. Eventually they may invade the overlying bone and stimulate osteoblastic activity causing new bone formation. A variety of histological patterns is described. The common pattern consists of whorls of spindle-shaped fibroblastic cells with concentrically laminated calcified bodies (psammoma bodies). Other meningiomas may appear more vascular. Sarcomatous change is rare.

Meningiomas present mostly in adult life and many are found coincidentally at post-mortem. Because they are attached to the dura and are well defined, these tumours may be successfully treated by surgery.

Nerve-sheath tumours

Neurofibroma

These tumours may be single or multiple (as in von Recklinghausen's disease). They arise on cranial, spinal and peripheral nerves, causing expansion of the nerve. They are usually ill-defined, merging with the surrounding connective tissue. Microscopically, neurofibromas consist of interlacing wavy bundles of delicate fibrils and Schwann cells. Vessels in the tumour are often hyalinized and there may be myxomatous change in the stroma.

Neurilemmoma

These tumours also may be single or multiple and associated with von Recklinghausen's disease (neurofibromatosis). They arise in the same distribution as neurofibromas. Those in the cranial nerves most commonly involve the eighth nerve and are called acoustic neuromas. Spinal tumours may protrude through the vertebral foramina as 'dumb-bell' tumours compressing spinal nerves. On peripheral nerves they may occur in the mediastinum or in the skin. Neurilemmomas are usually well circumscribed. They consist of bundles of fibrils and Schwann cells, the nuclei of which are arranged in rows or palisades. Myxomatous change in the tumour is common. These tumours are less liable to become malignant than neurofibromas.

Neurofibromatosis (von Recklinghausen's disease)

This is inherited as a Mendelian dominant. It is characterized by multiple neurofibromas and neurilemmomas, café-au-lait pigmentation of the skin, optic and cranial gliomas and meningiomas. There is a risk that one or more of these neurofibromas may undergo malignant change.

Neurofibrosarcoma

These tumours behave as fibrosarcomas, infiltrating locally and metastasizing by the bloodstream to the lungs. They may arise in preceding neurofibromas. Large deep-seated neurofibromas arising on main nerve trunks are more likely to become malignant than superficial tumours. Neurofibrosarcomas most often arise in the leg, posterior abdominal wall or thorax.

Neuroblastoma and ganglioneuroma

These tumours have been previously described (see p. 212).

26

The Skin

Inflammatory, allergic, traumatic and other 'medical' diseases of the skin form a specialized field in pathology and will not be considered in this chapter. Certain skin diseases are usually treated by surgical excision of the lesion or may be diagnosed by biopsy. It is these lesions which are seen most frequently in histopathology and which the student is more likely to see in histological sections.

Cysts

A cyst is a cavity lined by epithelium. *Sebaceous cysts* arise from hair follicles and are more accurately called *pilar cysts*. They are most commonly found on the scalp and are lined by stratified, plump eosinophilic epithelial cells which do not flatten near the cavity of the cyst. The cysts contain amorphous yellowish material which is eosinophilic. Occasionally, usually in women, tumours occur which have features in common with these cysts. The tumours may invade locally but they do not metastasize. Such tumours resemble squamous carcinoma and are referred to as pilar tumours (Cock's peculiar tumour). *Epidermoid cysts* are lined by stratified squamous epithelium and usually contain keratin. They may arise as a result of trauma, implanting epithelium in the dermis, or as a result of obstruction to the outflow from skin appendages. A *pilonidal cyst* is a form of epidermoid cyst occurring as a complication of a *pilonidal sinus*; these sinuses are usually found in the lower part of the back between the buttocks. Ingrowth of epidermis containing hairs may cause irritation and may become infected. Frequently the sinuses are found to track far out from the superficial punctum and wide excision is necessary to prevent recurrence. *Dermoid cysts* are developmental abnormalities and occur at lines of fusion of embryonic clefts. The angle of the eye or mouth is a common site. Histologically, dermoid cysts are similar to epidermoid cysts but their walls also contain well-formed skin adnexae.

Warts

The common wart, verruca vulgaris, occurs mainly in children but is also seen in adults. These warts are often multiple, especially on the hands.

Those that occur on the feet (plantar warts) become deeply embedded due to the pressure of weight-bearing and may be painful. Condylomata acuminata are warts which occur in the anogenital region and form large, fleshy outgrowths. All these warts are due to virus infection. The common wart consists of hyperplastic squamous epithelium (acanthosis) thrown in papillary folds (papillomatosis) and covered by thickened keratin (hyperkeratosis). Superficial cells in the epidermis become vacuolated and contain keratohyaline granules. Condylomata acuminata do not usually show so much hyperkeratosis and they may have an oedematous connective tissue core infiltrated by plasma cells.

Molluscum contagiosum is another viral infection of the skin resulting in umbilicated nodules a few millimetres in diameter. Histologically, it shows flask-shaped hyperplasia of squamous epithelium which contains characteristic inclusion bodies within some cells—molluscum bodies. Minor trauma is usually sufficient to cause a host reaction which destroys the lesion.

Keratoacanthoma, also known as molluscum sebaceum, may present as a rapidly growing wart or it may mimic squamous carcinoma. Keratoacanthoma arises on hair-bearing skin as a dome-shaped nodule with a central keratin plug. This wart may reach a size of 2 cm in the course of a few weeks but usually undergoes spontaneous regression in three to six months. In old people, regression is often incomplete and squamous carcinoma may develop. Histologically, keratoacanthoma shows epidermal proliferation with downgrowth of epithelium to form a hemispherical mass. There is surface keratinization to form the keratin plug seen macroscopically. The surrounding epidermis is normal; in this way keratoacanthoma differs from most squamous carcinomas which arise in a field of atypical squamous epithelium, often the result of solar irradiation (solar keratoses).

Seborrhoeic wart is more appropriately called a *basal cell papilloma*. These pigmented papillomas occur most frequently in elderly people anywhere on the skin surface other than the palms and soles. They show basal cell proliferation, characteristically raised above the level of the surrounding epidermis. Keratin cysts may form within the basal epithelium. Often there are features of similarity between basal cell papillomas and warty naevi (*naevus verrucosus*), the latter being foci of congenital papillary hyperplasia of the epidermis with overlying hyperkeratosis.

Premalignant conditions and carcinoma-in-situ

Irradiation by sunlight is the commonest predisposing factor in producing carcinoma in the skin. X-rays were an important cause in radiologists before the danger was recognized. Tar and certain mineral oils are also important, and there are still cases of skin cancer in elderly people due to taking arsenic in Fowler's solution for skin diseases or as a 'tonic' years ago.

Sunlight produces degeneration of dermal collagen so that it assumes some of the staining characteristics of elastin. The epidermis shows atypical squamous cells and abnormal formation of keratin resulting in *solar keratosis*. This is a premalignant change and squamous carcinoma often develops.

Some mucous membranes (e.g. buccal cavity, ectocervix) are covered with non-keratinizing stratified squamous epithelium. In some pathological situations, this epithelium keratinizes; the keratinized areas which are moist then appear white on naked-eyed examination and the term *leucoplakia* is often applied to them. Inflammatory, preneoplastic and neoplastic conditions can all give this appearance, so caution should be used with this term. It is better not to use this word, but to described the naked-eye appearance and more accurately classify the underlying epithelial abnormality.

Bowen's disease is a form of intraepidermal squamous cell carcinoma very similar to that produced by arsenic. There is gross atypia of the full thickness of the epidermis, with bizarre giant cells, abnormal mitoses and keratinization of individual cells. The lesions occur as single or multiple red plaques originally described on the trunk but occurring anywhere on the body surface.

Paget's disease of the nipple has been described in the chapter on breast diseases (see p. 203). Rarely, Paget's disease may occur in the anogenital and abdominal skin. Under these circumstances it may be associated with rectal or sebaceous carcinoma.

Basal cell carcinoma

This is probably the commonest malignant tumour in man. It does not metastasize and most are successfully treated so that very few cause death. These carcinomas may be single or multiple and arise in normal or solar-damaged skin. If untreated, basal cell carcinomas infiltrate and eventually erode surrounding structures including bone. Histologically, they consist of proliferating basal cells, usually in rounded islands invading the dermis. Less frequently, they may become cystic or pseudoglandular due to mucoid degeneration of dermal collagen. Some are pigmented and may mimic malignant melanoma.

Squamous cell carcinoma

Squamous carcinoma very rarely develops in skin which does not show evidence of one of the precancerous lesions already described. These carcinomas occur mainly on light-exposed areas; those that arise on the trunk are more often associated with arsenical keratoses. They may form a papillary mass or they may ulcerate. The rate of growth varies from case to case as does the degree of differentiation. Usually it is possible on microscopy to see keratinizing 'pearls' of squamous epithelium infiltrating the dermis. In other cases, differentiation may be so poor that the tumour cells are spindle shaped and mimic sarcoma.

Squamous carcinoma differs from basal cell carcinoma in its behaviour for untreated squamous carcinoma metastasizes, usually involving lymph nodes first.

Pigmented naevi and melanoma

Melanin is produced in the skin by melanocytes which are clear cells found in the basal layer of the epidermis. Melanin is passed from these cells to epithelial cells which, as a result, may appear pigmented. This accounts for the pigmentation seen in some basal cell papillomas and carcinomas. Melanocytes are probably of neuroectodermal origin and migrate from the neural crest to the skin. Some leave the epidermis and come to lie in the dermis as naevus cells. Dihydroxyphenylalanine (DOPA) is used as a substrate to demonstrate the presence of the enzyme tyrosinase which converts DOPA (and tyrosine) to melanin, and this enzyme is found only in the melanin-producing melanocyte. In pigmented skin, the melanocytes produce melanin which is then exported and is found in the cytoplasm of normal basal cells (melanophores).

A common *freckle (ephelis)* is a hyperpigmented area of skin which has a normal complement of melanocytes, though these may be hyperfunctioning. A *lentigo* is a hyperpigmented area of skin but with an increased number of melanocytes scattered regularly in its basal layer. Pigmented naevi are hamartomatous collections of naevus cells that may be found in the dermis or epidermis. The type commonly found in adults is entirely within the dermis—intradermal cellular naevus. It consists of nests of naevus cells which become gradually sclerosed in the deeper layers. Any pigment within them is confined to the superficial layers. Multinucleate giant cells may also be found in the superficial layers. In children, collections of naevus cells are more commonly found in the epidermis. These are known as junctional naevi. When groups of naevus cells are present at the junction and in the dermis, they are called compound naevi. Proliferation of naevus cells implies immaturity of the lesion and although this is acceptable in childhood and adolescence, it should be regarded with caution in adults. Cellular naevi in the palms and soles remain junctional throughout life. Blue naevi are pigmented fibroblastic lesions which occur deep in the dermis. It is this depth which makes the melanin appear blue. The naevus cells in blue naevi have not migrated to the epidermis and so do not assume the epithelioid features of cellular naevi. Blue naevi rarely become malignant; they are closely allied to Mongolian blue spot found in the lower part of the back in Mongolian races.

Malignant melanoma is a malignant tumour of melanocytes and accounts for half the deaths from malignant tumours of the skin. Some melanomas arise in long-standing cellular naevi, but others show no evidence of a preceding naevus. They may occur anywhere on the body surface but particularly on sun-exposed areas in pale-skinned people, though sites of friction and trauma are also important. The primary site may remain small and clinically undetected in spite of massive deposits of metastatic tumour. Most malignant melanomas are pigmented but some are amelanotic. Any recent increase in size of a pigmented skin lesion, especially if accompanied by ulceration and bleeding, should always be suspected as malignant melanoma. Histologically, malignant melanomas may show some features of similarity to cellular naevi but they show junctional activity, greater pleomorphism, bizarre tumour giant cells and frequent mitoses. Epidermal invasion carries tumour cells to the most superficial layers of the epidermis. On the deep aspect there is usually a lymphocytic infiltrate in the dermis. This probably represents a host immune reaction to the tumour and is of interest in view of the demonstration of serum antibodies to melanoma cells in patients with localized disease. Pigmented cells may be found at all layers and not confined to the surface as in cellular naevi. Lateral extension is very common and an important cause of recurrence following surgical excision. Malignant melanoma always requires excision of a wide zone of apparently normal surrounding skin. Lymphatic spread to regional lymph nodes and bloodstream spread to lungs and liver are common. The prognosis of malignant melanoma can be judged by measuring the thickness of the tumour—<0.75 mm has a good prognosis, >3 mm a bad prognosis—and the depth of invasion into the dermis and subcutaneous fat.

Not all malignant melanomas grow rapidly and metastasize early. Those that occur on the face in elderly people usually have a fairly good prognosis, but those on the hands and feet are much more sinister. Occasionally proliferation of melanoma cells is confined to the epidermis and is then known as a *malignant lentigo*. This may be regarded as in-situ melanoma. It does not metastasize until it invades the dermis.

Malignant melanoma is very uncommon before puberty and one should be wary of the diagnosis in the young. A benign pigmented lesion sometimes mistaken for malignant melanoma is Spitz naevus (juvenile melanoma). It is best regarded as a rather active compound naevus.

Dermal tumours

Dermatofibroma (histiocytoma, sclerosing haemangioma) is a common dermal 'tumour' that has many features of reactive rather than neoplastic proliferation. It is hard and smooth, producing a rounded swelling in the skin. Its cut surface appears yellow or cream coloured due to the presence of lipid-laden histiocytes. Various names are given to the lesion because at different stages of development vascular proliferation, histiocytic infiltration and fibrosis may be prominent features. Dermatofibromas are poorly circumscribed but benign.

Dermatofibrosarcoma protuberans is the malignant counterpart of dermatofibroma. It is a larger lesion and shows greater mitotic activity. There may be infiltration of underlying fat. Recurrence after attempted excision is common but these tumours rarely metastasize.

Leiomyoma may arise in the dermis from arrector pili muscles or from the wall of blood vessels. The latter is more common and gives rise to a rounded tender nodule in the deep dermis and subcutaneous fat.

Neurofibroma and *neurilemmoma* are both found in the skin; they have been described previously (see p. 249).

Glomus tumours are angiomatous malformations which are found in skin, where they cause small painful nodules. Histologically, they consist of vascular channels surrounded by glomus cells. These are small cells with clear cytoplasm, probably derived from pericytes. The lesions are richly supplied with nerves which probably accounts for the pain which is the most important clinical feature.

Other vascular malformations found in the dermis include haemangioma and lymphangioma. Rarely, angiosarcoma may arise in the skin, and then follows vascular obstruction, particularly to lymphatic vessels. Angiosarcomas are highly malignant neoplasms, metastasizing by the bloodstream. Multifocal primary angiosarcomas may be found in limbs with chronic lymphoedema. Kaposi's sarcoma presents with multiple skin plaques, usually in adults. Histologically, the lesions consist of proliferating blood vessels and spindle cells, the nature of which is uncertain. There may be haemosiderin pigmentation due to escape of blood from the small proliferating capillaries. Foci of similar tumours are found in internal organs in the aggressive form of the disease.

Further Reading

General and systemic

Larger undergraduate textbooks also used by postgraduates reading for higher diplomas. They have chapters on general pathology but also describe pathological changes affecting each of the body's organ systems.

Anderson, J.R (ed.) (1980) *Muir's Textbook of Pathology*, 11th ed. London: Edward Arnold.

Anderson, W.A.D. and Kissane, J.M. (1984) *Pathology*, 8th ed. St Louis, Mo: Mosby.

Robbins, S.L. and Cotran, R.S. (1984) *Pathologic Basis of Disease*, 3rd ed. Philadelphia: W.B. Saunders.

General pathology

Walter, J.B. and Israel, M.S. (1979) *General Pathology*, 5th ed. Edinburgh: Churchill Livingstone.

A very good account of general pathology originally written for surgeons reading for higher diplomas, but with a much wider appeal.

Systemic pathology

Symmers, W.St.C. (ed.) (1976–1980) *Systemic Pathology* (6 vols.), 2nd ed. Edinburgh: Churchill Livingstone.

A monumental work giving an account of pathological processes as they affect each organ system. Primarily written for histopathologists and with an emphasis on structural changes.

Index